Covid-19 Molecular Testing and Clinical Correlates

Editors

SANJAT KANJILAL
YI-WEI TANG

CLINICS IN LABORATORY MEDICINE

www.labmed.theclinics.com

Editor-In-Chief
MILENKO JOVAN TANASIJEVIC

June 2022 • Volume 42 • Number 2

ELSEVIER

1600 John F. Kennedy Boulevard • Suite 1800 • Philadelphia, Pennsylvania, 19103-2899

http://www.theclinics.com

CLINICS IN LABORATORY MEDICINE Volume 42, Number 2
June 2022 ISSN 0272-2712, ISBN-13: 978-0-323-84952-4

Editor: Katerina Heidhausen
Developmental Editor: Ann Gielou M. Posedio

Reprints. For copies of 100 or more, of articles in this publication, please contact the Commercial Reprints Department, Elsevier Inc., 360 Park Avenue South, New York, New York 10010-1710. Tel. 212-633-3874, Fax: 212-633-3820, E-mail: reprints@elsevier.com.

Clinics in Laboratory Medicine (ISSN 0272-2712) is published quarterly by Elsevier Inc., 360 Park Avenue South, New York, NY 10010-1710. Months of issue are March, June, September, and December. Business and Editorial offices: 1600 John F. Kennedy Blvd., Suite 1800, Philadelphia, PA 19103-2899. Periodicals postage paid at NewYork, NY and additional mailing offices. Subscription prices are $283.00 per year (US individuals), $753.00 per year (US institutions), $100.00 per year (US students), $363.00 per year (Canadian individuals), $776.00 per year (Canadian institutions), $100.00 per year (Canadian students), $404.00 per year (international individuals), $776.00 per year (international institutions), $185.00 (international students). Foreign air speed delivery is included in all Clinics subscription prices. All prices are subject to change without notice. POSTMASTER: Send address changes to *Clinics in Laboratory Medicine*, Elsevier Health Sciences Division, Subscription Customer Service, 3251 Riverport Lane, Maryland Heights, MO 63043. **Customer Service: 1-800-654-2452 (US). From outside of the US and Canada, call 1-314-447-8871. Fax: 1-314-447-8029. E-mail: journalscustomerservice-usa@elsevier.com (for print support) or journalsonlinesupport-usa@elsevier.com (for online support).**

Clinics in Laboratory Medicine is covered in *EMBASE/Exerpta Medica, MEDLINE/PubMed (Index Medicus), Cinahl, Current Contents/Clinical Medicine, BIOSIS and ISI/BIOMED.*

Contributors

EDITOR-IN-CHIEF

MILENKO JOVAN TANASIJEVIC, MD, MBA
Vice Chair for Clinical Pathology and Quality, Department of Pathology, Director of Clinical Laboratories, Brigham and Women's Hospital, Dana-Farber Cancer Institute, Associate Professor of Pathology, Harvard Medical School, Boston, Massachusetts, USA

EDITORS

SANJAT KANJILAL, MD, MPH
Department of Population Medicine, Harvard Medical School, Harvard Pilgrim Healthcare Institute, Boston, Massachusetts, USA; Division of Infectious Diseases, Brigham & Women's Hospital, Boston, Massachusetts, USA

YI-WEI TANG, MD, PhD
Medical Affairs, Danaher Diagnostic Platform/Cepheid, Shanghai, China

AUTHORS

SHAZAAD AHMAD, BMedSci, BMBS, MSc, FRCPath
Department of Virology, UK Health Security Agency, Manchester Foundation Trust, Manchester, United Kingdom

N. ESTHER BABADY, PhD, D(ABMM)
Member (Professor), Department of Pathology and Laboratory Medicine (Clinical Microbiology Services), Memorial Sloan Kettering Cancer Center (Infectious Disease Service), Department of Medicine, Memorial Sloan Kettering Cancer Center, New York, New York, USA

GAMA BANDAWE, PhD
Senior Lecturer, Head of Department, Biological Sciences Department, Academy of Medical Sciences, Malawi University of Science and Technology, Limbe, Malawi

JOSEPH BITILIYU-BANGOH, MSc
Deputy Director, Health Technical Support Services, Ministry of Health, Lilongwe, Malawi

MATTHEW J. BINNICKER, PhD, D(ABMM)
Director of Clinical Virology, Department of Laboratory Medicine and Pathology, Division of Clinical Microbiology, Mayo Clinic, Rochester, Minnesota, USA

ANDREW BIRTLES, BSc, MSc, PhD
Department of Virology, UK Health Security Agency, Manchester Foundation Trust, Manchester, United Kingdom

BENJAMIN BROWN, BSc, MSc, PhD
Department of Virology, UK Health Security Agency, Manchester Foundation Trust, Manchester, United Kingdom

SUSAN M. BUTLER-WU, PhD
Department of Pathology, Keck School of Medicine of USC, Los Angeles, California, USA

MICHELLE R. CAMPBELL, MS, MLS(ASCP)CMMBCM
Senior Developer, Department of Laboratory Medicine and Pathology, Translational Research, Innovation, and Test Development Office, Mayo Clinic, Rochester, Minnesota, USA

MOSES CHITENJE, BSc
Laboratory Officer, International Teaching and Education Centre for Health (I-TECH), Public Health Institute of Malawi, Ministry of Health, Lilongwe, Malawi

SANCHITA DAS, MD
Department of Laboratory Medicine, National Institutes of Health Clinical Center, Bethesda, Maryland, USA

EMMA DAVIES, BSc, MSc, DClinSci, FRCPath
Department of Virology, UK Health Security Agency, Manchester Foundation Trust, Manchester, United Kingdom

HAMZAH Z. FAROOQ, MBChB, MRCP, MSc, DipRCPath
Department of Virology, UK Health Security Agency, Department of Infectious Diseases and Tropical Medicine, North Manchester General Hospital, Manchester Foundation Trust, Manchester, United Kingdom

JENNIFER DIEN BARD, PhD, D(ABMM)
Director of Microbiology and Virology Laboratories, Department of Pathology and Laboratory Medicine, Children's Hospital Los Angeles, Associate Professor of Pathology, Keck School of Medicine of USC, Los Angeles, California, USA

KAREN M. FRANK, MD, PhD
Department of Laboratory Medicine, National Institutes of Health Clinical Center, Bethesda, Maryland, USA

MALCOLM GUIVER, BSc, PhD, FRCPath
Department of Virology, UK Health Security Agency, Manchester Foundation Trust, Manchester, United Kingdom

KIMBERLY E. HANSON, MD, MHS
ARUP Laboratories, Department of Medicine, Division of Infectious Diseases, University of Utah School of Medicine, Salt Lake City, Utah, USA

LOUISE HESKETH, BSc, PhD, FRCPath
Department of Virology, UK Health Security Agency, Manchester Foundation Trust, Manchester, United Kingdom

GARY L. HOROWITZ, MD
Department of Pathology and Laboratory Medicine, Tufts Medical Center, Tufts University School of Medicine, Boston, Massachusetts, USA

ELIZABETH KAMPIRA, PhD
Laboratory Adviser, Centres for Disease Control and Prevention, Lilongwe, Malawi

BENJAMIN KUKULL, MD
Department of Pathology, Cascade Pathology Services/Legacy Health, Portland, Oregon, USA

YANJUN LU, PhD
Associate professor, Department of Laboratory Medicine, Tongji Hospital, Tongji Medical College, Huazhong University of Science and Technology, Wuhan, China

NICHOLAS MACHIN, BMedSci, BMBS, MSc, FRCPath
Department of Virology, UK Health Security Agency, Manchester Foundation Trust, Manchester, United Kingdom

ALEXANDER J. McADAM, MD, PhD
Medical Director, Infectious Diseases Diagnostic Laboratory, Department of Laboratory Medicine, Boston Children's Hospital, Associate Professor of Pathology, Harvard Medical School, Boston, Massachusetts, USA

ASHLEY McEWAN, BSc, MSc
Department of Virology, UK Health Security Agency, Manchester Foundation Trust, Manchester, United Kingdom

ROBERT WILLIAM O'HARA, BSc, PGCert, MSc, PhD, FIBMS
Department of Virology, UK Health Security Agency, Manchester Foundation Trust, Manchester, United Kingdom

MATTHEW A. PETTENGILL, PhD, D(ABMM)
Assistant Professor, Director of Clinical Microbiology, Department of Pathology, Anatomy, and Cell Biology, Thomas Jefferson University, Philadelphia, Pennsylvania, USA

KYLE G. RODINO, PhD, D(ABMM)
Assistant Professor, Department of Pathology and Laboratory Medicine, Perelman School of Medicine, University of Pennsylvania, Assistant Director, Clinical Microbiology Laboratory, Hospital of the University of Pennsylvania, Philadelphia, Pennsylvania, USA

SALIKA M. SHAKIR, PhD
Department of Pathology, Section of Clinical Microbiology, University of Utah, School of Medicine, ARUP Laboratories, Salt Lake City, Utah, USA

KENNETH P. SMITH, PhD, D(ABMM)
Assistant Professor of Clinical Pathology and Laboratory Medicine, Perelman School of Medicine, University of Pennsylvania, Assistant Director, Infectious Disease Diagnostics Laboratory, Children's Hospital of Philadelphia, Philadelphia, Pennsylvania, USA

ZIYONG SUN, PhD
Professor, Department of Laboratory Medicine, Tongji Hospital, Tongji Medical College, Huazhong University of Science and Technology, Wuhan, China

PETER TILSTON, BSc, MSc
Department of Virology, UK Health Security Agency, Manchester Foundation Trust, Manchester, United Kingdom

NICOLE V. TOLAN, PhD, DABCC
Department of Pathology, Brigham and Women's Hospital, Harvard Medical School, Boston, Massachusetts, USA

THAO T. TRUONG, PhD
Department of Pathology and Laboratory Medicine, Children's Hospital Los Angeles, Los Angeles, California, USA

Contents

Caregivers may wish to use the Ct value to determine the progression of infection, how severe the infection will be, and whether the patient can transmit the virus. Variability of Ct values and the data supporting these uses should be considered when deciding whether and how to use Ct values in clinical care.

Nasopharyngeal swabs have historically been considered the preferred specimen type for the detection of respiratory viruses, including SARS-CoV-2. However, in response to a global pandemic with shortages of swabs and specimen transport media, limited access to qualified health care personnel, and needs for large-scale testing in nonmedical settings, alternative sample types have been validated for COVID-19 diagnosis. The purpose of this review is to highlight the diagnostic accuracy and clinical utility of non-nasopharyngeal respiratory samples for SARS-CoV-2 molecular diagnostic testing.

Scaling up SARS-CoV-2 testing during the COVID-19 pandemic was critical to maintaining clinical operations and an open society. Pooled testing and automation were two critical strategies used by laboratories to meet the unprecedented demand. Here, we review these and other cutting-edge strategies that sought to expand SARS-CoV-2 testing capacity while maintaining high individual test performance.

Deployment of molecular testing for SARS-CoV-2 in resource-limited settings is challenging. Scale-up of molecular had to be conducted with a laboratory system strengthening approach that emphasize laboratory integration. National reference laboratories play a central role. In Malawi the molecular testing was underpinned by existing pathogen control programs for human immunodeficiency virus and tuberculosis that use Abbott and GeneXpert machines and reagents. Despite this, the impact on these programs was well managed. Antigen testing increased access to testing. Pooled testing and direct-to-polymerase chain reaction methods have the potential to save costs and further increase access to molecular tests.

From the onset of the severe acute respiratory syndrome coronavirus 2 (SARS-CoV-2)/COVID-19 pandemic, there has been a major emphasis on molecular laboratory tests for the virus. Shortages in various testing supplies, the desire to increase testing capacity, and a push to make point-of-care or home-based testing available have fostered considerable innovation for SARS-CoV-2 molecular diagnostics, advancements likely to be applicable to other diagnostic uses. The authors attempt to cover some of the most compelling novel types of molecular assays or novel approaches in adapting established molecular methodologies for SARS-CoV-2 detection or characterization.

CLINICS IN LABORATORY MEDICINE

SERIES OF RELATED INTEREST

Surgical Pathology Clinics
Available at: https://www.surgpath.theclinics.com/

THE CLINICS ARE NOW AVAILABLE ONLINE!
Access your subscription at:
www.theclinics.com

Preface

A Tale of Trial and Triumph: Molecular Diagnostics for Severe Acute Respiratory Coronavirus 2 Over the First Two Years of the Coronavirus Disease 2019 Pandemic

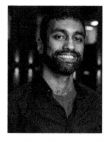
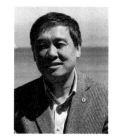

Sanjat Kanjilal, MD, MPH   Yi-Wei Tang, MD, PhD
Editors

Without doubt, the coronavirus disease 2019 (COVID-19) pandemic has been the most serious health crisis to impact the world since the 1918 influenza pandemic. At the time of this writing, there are nearly 432 million documented cases, 5.9 million deaths, and an untold number of people suffering from chronic symptoms.[1] COVID-19 is caused by an infection from the severe acute respiratory syndrome coronavirus 2 (SARS-CoV-2), a single-stranded, positive-sense, enveloped RNA virus of the sarbecovirus subgenus that is transmitted primarily through respiratory droplets.

Diagnosis of SARS-CoV-2 infection is one of the 4 pillars of COVID-19 pandemic control, alongside nonpharmacologic interventions, vaccination, and genomic surveillance. Despite years of experience with molecular diagnostics for respiratory viruses, laboratories across the world faced an unprecedented challenge in having to rapidly build, scale, and diversify SARS-CoV-2 testing capacity. Some of these challenges were due to the virus itself, including its penchant for transmission from asymptomatic carriers and its ability to evolve under immune selective pressure. However, other equally challenging problems were due to crippling supply

Clin Lab Med 42 (2022) xiii–xv
https://doi.org/10.1016/j.cll.2022.04.001
0272-2712/22/© 2022 Published by Elsevier Inc.

chain issues, and a regulatory infrastructure ill equipped to handle a fast-moving emergency.

In this issue of *Clinics in Laboratory Medicine*, we have assembled a series of articles that provide a comprehensive overview of the state of SARS-CoV-2 molecular testing two years into the COVID-19 pandemic. Our intention is to provide readers deep insight into the experiences of clinical laboratories around the world, written by leading experts with first-hand experience from the frontlines. We cover a diverse set of topics ranging from detailed looks at the major commercial molecular assays deployed in the United States (articles in this issue, "Analytic and Clinical Performance of Major Commercial SARS-CoV-2 Molecular Assays in the United States" by Campbell and Binnicker and "The Successes and Challenges of SARS-CoV-2 Molecular Testing in the United States" by Bard), Europe ("An Overview of SARS-CoV-2 Molecular Assays in Europe" by Davies and colleagues), and Asia ("SARS-CoV-2 Molecular Diagnostics in China" by Sun and Lu and online article by Heueh), to the benefits and pitfalls of testing at the point of care, in the form of either rapid antigen detection tests ("Rapid Antigen Assays for SARS-CoV-2: Promise and Peril" by Truong and colleagues) or molecular assays ("Point-of-Care Molecular Assays for SARS-CoV-2" by Tolan and Horowitz). We discuss the use of cycle threshold values for clinical decision making, as this is a completely novel use of respiratory viral diagnostics that has now become routine practice at many institutions ("Cycle Threshold Values from SARS-CoV-2 PCR Assays: Interpretation and Potential Use Cases" by McAdam). In addition, a key aspect of pandemic control is the ability to conduct mass testing; thus, we present a pair of articles that discuss the performance of alternative specimen types ("Performance of Nonnasopharyngeal Sample Types for Molecular Detection SARS-CoV-2" by Kukull and colleagues) and strategies used by labs to scale up their capacity ("Strategies for Scaling Up SARS-CoV-2 Molecular Testing Capacity" by Das and Frank). As disparities in access to SARS-CoV-2 testing have been a serious issue throughout the pandemic, we include a review of the many challenges with validating and scaling up testing in underresourced regions of the world ("Approaches to Deployment of Molecular Testing for SARS-CoV-2 in Resource-Limited Settings" by Bandawe). Finally, we present an overview of next-generation diagnostics that seek to overcome the problems of our existing technologies ("Novel Assays for Molecular Detection of SARS-CoV-2" by Pettengill and colleagues), an area of intense research and a silver lining hidden in this crisis.

SARS-CoV-2 is the third coronavirus to enter circulation in human populations in the past 20 years. With climate change, increasing encroachment into animal reservoirs, and world travel, it is nearly certain that we will experience another global pandemic in our lifetime. Thus, it is incumbent upon us to learn from the innumerable failures and successes of SARS-CoV-2 testing over the past two years, as we will undoubtably rely on this important knowledge base the next time the world faces a global health emergency.

Sanjat Kanjilal, MD, MPH
Department of Population Medicine
Harvard Medical School
Harvard Pilgrim Healthcare Institute
Boston, MA, USA

Division of Infectious Diseases, Brigham & Women's Hospital
Boston, MA USA

Yi-Wei Tang, MD, PhD
Medical Affairs
Danaher Diagnostic Platform/Cepheid
518 Fuquan North Road
Shanghai 200325, China

E-mail addresses:
skanjilal@bwh.harvard.edu (S. Kanjilal)
yi-wei.tang@cepheid.com (Y.-W. Tang)

REFERENCE

1. Johns Hopkins Coronavirus Resource Center. 2020. COVID-19 Map – Johns Hopkins Coronavirus Resource Center. Available at: https://coronavirus.jhu.edu/map.html. Accessed February 24, 2022.

Analytic and Clinical Performance of Major Commercial Severe Acute Respiratory Syndrome Coronavirus 2 Molecular Assays in the United States

Michelle R. Campbell, MS, MLS(ASCP)^CM MB^CM a,
Matthew J. Binnicker, PhD, D(ABMM)^b,*

KEYWORDS

- COVID-19 • SARS-CoV-2 • Emergency use authorization • Molecular
- Analytical sensitivity • Analytical specificity • Clinical performance

KEY POINTS

- Molecular assays to detect SARS-CoV-2 have been rapidly developed in response to the COVID-19 pandemic.
- Comparing the analytical and clinical performance of major commercial SARS-CoV-2 molecular assays provides an objective means of evaluating accuracy before implementation.
- With rare exceptions, molecular assays for the detection of SARS-CoV-2 offer comparable analytical and clinical performance.
- The lessons learned from the COVID-19 pandemic can be applied to the development and implementation of laboratory diagnostics in future outbreaks of novel infectious diseases.

INTRODUCTION

The global coronavirus disease 2019 (COVID-19) pandemic, caused by severe acute respiratory syndrome coronavirus 2 (SARS-CoV-2), has resulted in more than 276 million cases worldwide and greater than 51 million cases in the United States

^a Department of Laboratory Medicine and Pathology, Translational Research, Innovation, and Test Development Office, Mayo Clinic, 200 1st Street SW – Hilton 4-76, Rochester, MN 55905, USA; ^b Department of Laboratory Medicine and Pathology, Division of Clinical Microbiology, Mayo Clinic, 200 1st Street SW – Hilton 4-54, Rochester, MN 55905, USA
* Corresponding author.
E-mail address: binnicker.matthew@mayo.edu
Twitter: @DrMattBinnicker (M.J.B.)

Clin Lab Med 42 (2022) 129–145
https://doi.org/10.1016/j.cll.2022.02.001
0272-2712/22/© 2022 Elsevier Inc. All rights reserved.

alone.[1,2] With the rapid spread of the virus, the availability of clinical diagnostics to quickly and accurately detect SARS-CoV-2 has been essential to identify positive cases, manage patient care, and guide state and national response plans. To address the need for widescale testing, diagnostic test manufacturers and clinical laboratories have partnered to develop and implement molecular assays at an unprecedented pace. Increasing the testing capabilities in the United States has been facilitated by the issuance of emergency use authorizations (EUAs) by the U.S. Food and Drug Administration (FDA). Molecular diagnostic tests have been the primary means of diagnosing COVID-19, and at the time of preparing this article, greater than 200 SARS-CoV-2 molecular diagnostic tests have received EUA.[3] However, as the number of commercially available SARS-CoV-2 molecular assays has increased, so has the need to understand the differences between these methods. This review compares the analytical and clinical performance of major SARS-CoV-2 molecular assays available in the United States and suggests future topics for consideration.

OVERVIEW OF SEVERE ACUTE RESPIRATORY SYNDROME CORONAVIRUS 2 MOLECULAR ASSAYS
Selection of Assays

Commercially available SARS-CoV-2 molecular assays were included in this review if they were (1) listed in the 2021 College of American Pathologists' (CAP) Quality Cross Check: SARS-CoV-2 Molecular Program COV2Q-A Participant Summary, and (2) ≥20 participating laboratories were listed as using the method in the CAP summary.[4,5] The assays meeting these criteria are summarized in **Table 1**. The FDA maintains a complete list of individual EUAs for SARS-CoV-2 molecular diagnostic tests on its website.[3] Multiplexed panels were out of scope for this review.

Table 1
Major commercial SARS-CoV-2 molecular assays classified by turnaround time and throughput

Classification	Assay (Manufacturer)
Rapid/POC[a]	ID NOW COVID-19 (Abbott Diagnostics Scarborough, Inc., Scarborough, ME) Xpert Omni SARS-CoV-2 (Cepheid, Sunnyvale, CA) Xpert Xpress SARS-CoV-2 test (Cepheid)
Sample-to-answer[b]	BD SARS-CoV-2 Reagents for BD MAX System (Becton, Dickinson and Company [BD], Franklin Lakes, NJ) BioGX SARS-CoV-2 Reagents for BD MAX System (BD) BioFire COVID-19 Test (BioFire Defense, LLC, Salt Lake City, UT) Simplexa COVID-19 Direct assay (DiaSorin Molecular LLC, Cypress, CA) ePlex SARS-CoV-2 Test (GenMark Diagnostics, Inc., Carlsbad, CA) ARIES SARS-CoV-2 Assay (Luminex Corporation, Austin, TX) TaqPath COVID-19 Combo Kit (Thermo Fisher Scientific, Inc., Waltham, MA)
High-throughput[c]	Abbott RealTime SARS-CoV-2 assay (Abbott Molecular, Des Plaines, IL) Aptima SARS-CoV-2 assay (Hologic, Inc., Marlborough, MA) Panther Fusion SARS-CoV-2 Assay (Hologic) cobas SARS-CoV-2 (Roche Molecular Systems, Inc., Pleasanton, CA) Amplitude Solution with the TaqPath COVID-19 High-Throughput Combo Kit (Thermo Fisher Scientific)

Abbreviations: POC, point-of-care; TAT, turnaround time.
[a] TAT of ≤1 h; often single-sample throughput.
[b] TAT of ~1 to 4 h; throughput of up to several dozen samples/run.
[c] TAT of >3 to 4 h; throughput of greater than 450 samples/run.

Once molecular SARS-CoV-2 assays were identified for inclusion, they were further divided into one of the following 3 categories, similar to those applied by Fung and colleagues: (1) rapid/point-of-care (POC), (2) sample-to-answer, and (3) high-throughput.[6] Rapid/POC assays were those with a turnaround time (TAT) of ≤1 hour, the capability to be performed in a setting with a Clinical Laboratory Improvement Amendments (CLIA) Certificate of Waiver, and having a typical throughput of 1 sample/run.[3,7] Sample-to-answer platforms were those with a TAT of approximately 1 to 4 hours and a capacity to run several dozen samples/run. The final category consisted of assays performed using a high-throughput platform with the capacity to run more than 450 samples/day, but a typical TAT of greater than 3 to 4 hours (see **Table 1**).[3]

Molecular Technologies

To date, most SARS-CoV-2 molecular assays have used real-time reverse transcription–polymerase chain reaction (RT-PCR) technology. However, additional molecular technologies including transcription-mediated amplification (TMA), nested PCR, reverse transcription loop-mediated isothermal amplification (RT-LAMP), or RT-PCR with electrochemical detection have also been developed (**Table 2**).[3]

Molecular Targets

Molecular assays for the detection of SARS-CoV-2 often include greater than 1 gene target. Common targets include the RNA-dependent RNA polymerase (RdRp), nucleocapsid phosphoprotein (N), spike glycoprotein (S), small envelope protein (E), and open reading frame (ORF) genes. Of the assays included in this review, 6 target a single gene, whereas the remainder target ≥2 genes (see **Table 2**).[8–23]

Acceptable Specimen Types

Nasopharyngeal (NP) swabs in viral transport media or phosphate-buffered saline have been considered the gold-standard specimen type throughout the COVID-19 pandemic, and NP swabs are considered acceptable for all assays included in this review. In addition to NP swabs, many assays allow for other upper respiratory swab specimens to be tested, including oropharyngeal, nasal, and midturbinate swabs. A full list of acceptable specimen types are included in **Table 2**.[9,16,24–37]

ANALYTICAL PERFORMANCE
Analytical Sensitivity

Limit of detection
The analytical sensitivity (ie, limit of detection [LoD]) of a molecular assay is the lowest concentration of a target that can be detected in at least 19 (95%) of 20 replicates, as defined by the FDA Molecular Diagnostic Template for Commercial Manufacturers.[38] The manufacturers' established LoDs of major commercial SARS-CoV-2 molecular assays are summarized in **Table 3**. Although it is not possible to directly compare LoDs across all SARS-CoV-2 tests because of varying reporting units (eg, copies/mL vs genomic equivalents/mL), the analytical sensitivity varies across commercially available tests. Among assays with analytical sensitivity reported in copies/mL, the manufacturer's established LoD ranges from ∼30 copies/mL (cobas SARS-CoV-2) to 750–1000 copies/mL (ePlex SARS-CoV-2).[9,11,13,14,16,17,21,39,40]

Several groups have evaluated these methods and performed independent studies to confirm the LoD against the manufacturers' claims. In many studies, the LoDs were confirmed to be at or below the analytical sensitivity defined by the manufacturer.[6,41–55] Exceptions included the ID NOW COVID-19 and the TaqPath COVID-19

Table 2
Overview of major commercial SARS-CoV-2 molecular assays in the United States[3,8–21,24–37,39,40,84]

Assay	Platforms	Method	Gene Target(s)	Approved Specimen(s)
ID NOW COVID-19	ID NOW Instrument	RT, Isothermal amplification	RdRp	Nasal, NP, throat swabs
Abbott RealTime SARS-CoV-2 assay	Abbott m2000 System	Real-time RT-PCR	RdRp, N	NP, OP, nasal swabs; BAL
BD SARS-CoV-2 Reagents for BD MAX System	BD MAX System	Real-time RT-PCR	N1, N2	NP, anterior nasal, MT, OP swabs; NP wash/aspirate, nasal aspirates
BioGX SARS-CoV-2 Reagents for BD MAX BD MAX System System		Real-time RT-PCR	N1, N2	NP, OP swabs
BioFire COVID-19 Test	FilmArray 2.1 and FilmArray Torch Instrument Systems	RT, Nested multiplex PCR	ORF1ab[a], ORF8	NP, OP, midturbinate, anterior nasal swabs; sputum, endotracheal aspirate, BAL or mini-BAL
Xpert Omni SARS-CoV-2	GeneXpert Omni System	Real-time RT-PCR	E, N2	NP, OP, anterior nasal, MT swabs; nasal wash/aspirate
Xpert Xpress SARS-CoV-2 test	GeneXpert Dx and GeneXpert Infinity Systems	Real-time RT-PCR	E, N2	NP, OP, anterior nasal, MT swabs; nasal wash/aspirate
Simplexa COVID-19 Direct assay	LIAISON MDX	Real-time RT-PCR	ORF1ab, S	NP, anterior nasal swabs; nasal wash/aspirate, BAL
ePlex SARS-CoV-2 Test	ePlex instrument	RT-PCR and electrochemical detection	N[a]	NP swabs
Aptima SARS-CoV-2 assay	Panther and Panther Fusion systems	TMA, chemiluminescent	ORF1ab[a]	NP, OP, anterior nasal, MT swabs; NP wash/aspirate, nasal aspirate
Panther Fusion SARS-CoV-2 Assay	Panther Fusion System	Real-time RT-PCR	ORF1ab[a]	NP, OP, MT, nasal swabs; NP wash/aspirate, nasal wash, BAL
ARIES SARS-CoV-2 Assay	ARIES instrument	RT-PCR	ORF1ab, N	NP swabs
cobas SARS-CoV-2	cobas 6800 and 8800 Systems	Real-time RT-PCR	ORF1 a/b, E	NP, OP, nasal swabs; self-collected anterior nasal (nasal) swabs

| Amplitude Solution with the TaqPath COVID-19 High-Throughput Combo Kit | "Authorized real-time PCR instrument" | Real-time RT-PCR | Orf1ab, S, N | NP and anterior nasal swabs |
| TaqPath COVID-19 Combo Kit | "Authorized real-time PCR instrument" | Real-time RT-PCR | Orf1ab, S, N | NP, OP, MT, nasal swabs; NP aspirate, BAL, self-collected nasal swabs |

Abbreviations: BAL, bronchoalveolar lavage; E, small envelope; MT, midturbinate; N, nucleocapsid phosphoprotein; NP, nasopharyngeal; OP, oropharyngeal; Orf/ORF, open reading frame; PCR, polymerase chain reaction; RdRp, RNA-dependent RNA polymerase; RT, reverse transcription; S, spike glycoprotein; TMA, transcription-mediated amplification.

[a] Targets in 2 regions of a single gene.

Table 3
Analytical and clinical performance of major SARS-CoV-2 molecular assays[3,6,8–21,39–55,57–62,64,65]

Assay	Analytical Performance				Clinical Performance				Reference(s)
	Analytical Sensitivity (LoD)		Analytical Specificity (Cross-Reactivity) (Observed, Y/N)		Positive Percent Agreement		Negative Percent Agreement		
	Claimed	Observed	Claimed	Observed	Claimed	Observed	Claimed	Observed	
ID NOW COVID-19	125 GE/mL	262–20,000 copies/mL	N	NA	100%	48%–94%	100%	98.4%–100%	Abbott; Cradic et al,[57] 2020; Dinnes et al,[58] 2020; Fung et al,[6] 2020; Lee & Song,[65] 2021; Lephart, et al,[41] 2021; Mitchell & George,[59] 2020; Rhoads et al,[60] 2020; Zhen et al,[42] 2020
Abbott RealTime SARS-CoV-2 assay	100 copies/mL	32–53 copies/mL	N	N	100%	93%–96%	100%	100%	Degli-Angeli et al,[43] 2020; Fung et al,[6] 2020; Lephart et al,[41] 2021
BD SARS-CoV-2 Reagents for BD MAX System	640 GC/mL	251 copies/mL	N	NA	100%	100%	97%	96.7%	Yanson et al,[44] 2021
BioGX SARS-CoV-2 Reagents for BD MAX System	40 GE/mL	NA	N	NA	100%	NA	100%	NA	NA
BioFire COVID-19 Test	330 GC/mL	125–165 copies/mL 500 GE/mL	N	NA	90%–100%[a]	98.7%–100%	100%	100%	Eckbo et al,[46] 2021; Smith et al,[45] 2020
Xpert Omni SARS-CoV-2	400 copies/mL	NA	Y[b]	NA	100%	NA	100%	NA	NA
Xpert Xpress SARS-CoV-2 test	0.0200 PFU/mL	0.01 PFU/mL 8.26–100 copies/mL	Y[b]	Y[c]	97.8%	98.3%–100%	95.6%	95.8%–100%	Dinnes, et al,[58] 2020; Lephart et al,[41] 2021; Loeffelholz, et al,[47] 2020; Wolters et al,[48] 2020; Zhen et al,[42] 2020
Simplexa COVID-19 Direct assay	500 copies/mL[d]	39 ± 23–521 copies/mL	Y[e]	N	96.7%–100%[f]	88%–100%	100%	95.5%–100%	Bordi et al,[50] 2020; Cradic, et al,[57] 2020; Fung et al,[6] 2020; Lephart, et al,[41] 2021; Rhoads et al,[60]2020; Zhen et al,[49] 2020; Zhen et al,[42] 2020

Assay	LoD	Reaction range			PPA	PPA range	NPA	NPA range	References
ePlex SARS-CoV-2 Test	750–1000 copies/mL[g]	100–1000 copies/mL	Y[h]	NA	94.4%	91.4%–100%	100%	100%	Fung, et al.[6] 2020; Uhteg et al,[51] 2020; Zhen et al,[49] 2020; Zhen et al,[42] 2020
Aptima SARS-CoV-2 assay	0.01 TCID$_{50}$/mL	0.01–0.003 TCID$_{50}$/mL 62.5–612 copies/mL 500 GE/mL	N	N	100%	94.7%–100%	98.2%	98.7%–100%	Pham et al,[52] 2020; Schneider et al,[53] 2021; Smith et al,[45] 2020; Yanson et al,[44] 2021
Panther Fusion SARS-CoV-2 Assay	0.01 TCID$_{50}$/mL	62.5–100 copies/mL 1000 GE/mL	N	NA	100%	98.7%–100%	100%	96%–100%	Fung et al,[6] 2020; Smith et al,[45] 2020; Zhen et al,[49] 2020
ARIES SARS-CoV-2 Assay	180,000 NDU/mL	1000–10,000 copies/reaction range	N	NA	100%[i]	26.7%–100%	100%	100%	Lee et al,[62] 2021; Tanida et al,[54] 2020
cobas SARS-CoV-2	25–46 copies/mL[j]	≤ 10–298 copies/mL	N	NA	100%	94.2%–100%	100%	90%–100%	Cradic et al,[57] 2020; Fung et al,[6] ; Lee et al,[62] 2021; Pujadas et al,[64] 2020; Yanson et al,[44] 2021
Amplitude Solution with the TaqPath COVID-19 High-Throughput Combo Kit	250 GCE/mL[k]	NA	Y[l]	NA	100%	NA	100%	NA	NA
TaqPath COVID-19 Combo Kit	10 GCE/reaction	767 GC/mL	Y[l]	NA	100%	85.3%–100%	100%	70%–100%	Lee et al,[62] 2021; Matsumura et al,[55] 2021

Abbreviations: GC, genomic copies; GCE, genome copy equivalents; GE, genomic equivalents; LoD, limit of detection; N, no; NA, information not available; NDU, nucleic acid amplification test-detectable units; PFU, plaque-forming unit; TCID$_{50}$, median tissue culture infectious dose; Y, yes.

a Varies depending on the method of evaluation (eg, contrived vs clinical samples).
b E primers and probes will detect human SARS-CoV.
c E primers and probe detected SARS-CoV, resulting in a presumptive positive test result.
d Specific to nasopharyngeal swabs.
e Primer and/or probe sequence homology with SARS-CoV detected by in silico analysis, not observed during laboratory testing.
f Varies depending on specimen type.
g Varies depending on workflow used (with vs without sample delivery device).
h Primer and/or probe sequence homology with SARS-CoV by in silico analysis, also observed in laboratory testing.
i Overall PPA (PPA varies for individual gene targets).
j Varies depending on the target and method of analysis.
k Only confirmed through bridging study.
l Primer and/or probe sequence homology for N gene with *Neisseria elongata*. Given low homology with N gene reverse primer and probe, the risk for nonspecific amplification was determined to be low. Primer and/or probe sequence homology was also identified for "different isolates of the same species" (eg, strains of *Bacillus anthracis*), but amplification was deemed unlikely to occur.

Combo Kit, both of which demonstrated higher LoDs (262–20,000 and 767 copies/mL, respectively) during independent evaluations.[6,41,42,55] Of the rapid/POC assays, several studies have demonstrated that the Xpert Xpress SARS-CoV-2 test showed superior sensitivity (~10–100 copies/mL) compared with the ID NOW COVID-19 assay (262–20,000 copies/mL).[6,41,42,47,55] Independent studies generally confirmed the claimed analytical sensitivity of sample-to-answer assays, which range from approximately 40 to 1000 copies/mL. In contrast to several other sample-to-answer assays, the ePlex SARS-CoV-2 test has been shown to inconsistently detect samples with lower viral concentrations than the manufacturer's claimed LoD of 750 to 1000 copies/mL. Zhen and colleagues demonstrated that at concentrations of 1000 and 500 copies/mL, a decrease was noted in percent detected from 100% to 70%.[49] All high-throughput assays demonstrated excellent analytical sensitivity, with a study by Fung and colleagues determining the LoD for the cobas SARS-CoV-2 assay to be ≤ 10 copies/mL.[6] Yanson and colleagues established a higher LoD for this assay at 298 copies/mL, although details for the lowest concentration tested were unavailable and the LoDs determined for other assays (eg, Aptima SARS-CoV-2 assay) were also significantly higher (≥4 times) than observed in other studies.[44,45,52,53]

Inclusivity
Inclusivity studies can be performed by *in silico* analysis with the purpose of identifying the sequences that will be detected by the assay. Per FDA guidance, assays should detect 100% of SARS-CoV-2 strains, with a required risk assessment describing the potential impact on assay performance should sequences with less than 100% homology be identified during inclusivity studies.[38] Of the reviewed assays, a small number of manufacturers evaluated inclusivity by performing laboratory testing in addition to *in silico* analysis. Manufacturers claimed 86.4% to 100% alignment of oligonucleotide primer and probe sequences with SARS-CoV-2 sequences available in public databases, such as NCBI and GenBank. No manufacturers predicted an impact on the ability of their assay to detect published SARS-CoV-2 strains, including those with less than 100% alignment with available SARS-CoV-2 sequences.[8–21,39,40] It must be noted that reported coverage will vary based on the number of sequences available for comparison at the time the *in silico* analysis is performed. This is especially important as new variants of SARS-CoV-2 emerge.

Analytical Specificity

Cross-reactivity
The analytical specificity of molecular diagnostics can be evaluated through cross-reactivity studies. The purpose of these studies is to ensure that the molecular assay does not react with similar, potentially related pathogens or other organisms that may be present in clinical specimens. The FDA provides a list of recommended organisms to include in cross-reactivity studies by *in silico* analysis and laboratory testing. This includes other members of the family *Coronaviridae* (eg, human coronaviruses 229E, OC43, HKU1, NL63, SARS-CoV, and MERS-CoV) as well as organisms that are likely to be present in respiratory specimens. Recommendations are provided for follow-up studies should significant homology (>80%) with a potential cross-reactive sequence be identified.[38]

Table 3 summarizes the results of cross-reactivity studies and *in silico* analyses performed by manufacturers to ensure analytical specificity. Multiple manufacturers reported the potential for cross-reactivity with coronaviruses known to infect animals (eg, bat and pangolin coronaviruses) as well as SARS-CoV, which is not unexpected because of high genetic homology with SARS-CoV-2. No manufacturers noted cross-reactivity with MERS-CoV or other organisms likely to be present in respiratory samples.[8,10–21,39,40,56] Independent evaluation of commercial assays has not revealed significant cross-reactivity that would raise concern for false-positive results because of the presence of nonspecific sequences.[43,47,50,52]

CLINICAL PERFORMANCE
Percent Agreement

In addition to analytical studies, the clinical performance must also be evaluated when developing molecular assays for SARS-CoV-2. The FDA recommends calculating positive percent agreement (PPA) in comparison to a high sensitivity EUA RT-PCR test. Furthermore, it is recommended that the comparator assay uses an "internationally recognized standard" or the FDA's SARS-CoV-2 Reference Panel to establish the sensitivity of the assay. Recommendations for assessing the agreement of negative results (ie, negative percent agreement [NPA]) are comparison with an EUA RT-PCR test using prospectively collected samples or "as agreement with expected results if samples were collected from individuals known to be negative for SARS-CoV-2 (eg, collected before December 2019)." The comparator EUA RT-PCR does not need to have identical targets to the assay being evaluated. The acceptance criteria for positive and negative agreement is $\geq$ 95%.[38]

Table 3 summarizes available information on clinical performance, as demonstrated by PPA and NPA between methods. Manufacturer claims for overall PPA ranged from 90% to 100%.[8–21,39,40] The ARIES SARS-CoV-2 assay demonstrated only 25% to 40% agreement for the ORF1ab target, but 100% agreement for the N target; however, only 1 of the 2 targets must be detected for the assay result to be interpreted as positive.[18] During independent evaluations, the observed PPA for most commercial assays was similar to manufacturer claims with the exception of the ID NOW COVID-19 device and ARIES SARS-CoV-2 assay, which both claimed 100% PPA and demonstrated PPA ranging from 48% to 94% and 26.7% to 100% in published studies, respectively.[41,42,54,57–62] Possible explanations for the differences observed with the ID NOW COVID-19 PPA may be variations in the comparator assays and the fact that the manufacturer evaluated PPA at 2 to 5 times the LoD, while the referenced studies may have included samples with lower viral loads.[10] The study that determined the ARIES SARS-CoV-2 assay PPA to be 26.7% was based on comparison with the Xpert Xpress SARS-CoV-2 as the reference method and specifically evaluated weakly positive samples (ie, Ct > 34 in the Xpert Xpress SARS-CoV2 assay). When only strongly positive samples (ie, Ct < 34 for at least one target gene in the Xpert Xpress SARS-CoV2 assay) were included in the analysis, PPA increased to 100%.[54] Manufacturer claims for NPA ranged from 95.6% to 100%.[8–16,18–21,39,40,63] Most observed NPAs were similar to manufacturer claims, with the exception of the TaqPath COVID-19 Combo Kit, for which a single study observed 70% NPA based on consensus of 4 molecular assays.[41–45,47,49,50,53,57,58,61,62,64,65]

Comparison with Clinical Evaluation

Although the "gold standard" for the diagnosis of SARS-CoV-2 infections is molecular testing, there is limited information on the clinical performance of these assays through comparison with clinical findings and radiologic evidence of COVID-19.[66,67] In particular, chest computerized tomography (CT) has been suggested as a complementary diagnostic test for patients with suspected SARS-CoV-2 infection.[68] Studies in which patients underwent both RT-PCR testing and chest CT imaging suggest that chest CT is highly sensitive for the diagnosis of SARS-CoV-2 infection and can identify likely cases of SARS-CoV-2 that were missed by RT-PCR. Two studies of patients in Wuhan, China, demonstrated 97% sensitivity of chest CT using positive RT-PCR results as the reference standard.[68,69] In another study, an in-depth evaluation of 5 patients with initial negative SARS-CoV-2 RT-PCR was performed and showed that chest CT findings were consistent with a SARS-CoV-2 infection before a positive RT-PCR result.[70] Although studies directly evaluating SARS-CoV-2 RT-PCR results with imaging studies and other clinical/epidemiologic findings are few in number, there are now published data showing that in patients with COVID-19 (ie, as determined by clinical and/or radiology findings), SARS-CoV-2 molecular testing may need to be performed multiple times, or on alternate sample types (eg, bronchoalveolar lavage fluid) to yield a positive result.[66,68,70]

It has also been demonstrated that the sensitivity of commercially available molecular assays may depend on when testing is performed during the course of disease. Theoretically, tests detecting SARS-CoV-2 RNA will have the lowest false-negative rate when the viral load is at its highest. He and colleagues proposed that peak viral loads occur around the time of symptom onset, which is typically 3 to 5 days post-exposure.[66,71] This suggests that rapid/POC tests, such as the Xpert Xpress SARS-CoV-2 and ID NOW COVID-19 tests, are likely to provide the highest negative predictive value when performed in symptomatic patients who are early in their disease course. As the clinical course progresses and viral load decreases, the risk for false-negative results increases and using an assay with the lowest (ie, best) analytical sensitivity becomes increasingly important.

DISCUSSION

Although the rapid development and implementation of molecular assays to detect SARS-CoV-2 has addressed the acute need for diagnostic tools during the COVID-19 pandemic, there are remaining questions to consider. Of particular concern is whether currently available molecular assays will continue to detect emerging SARS-CoV-2 variants. The World Health Organization (WHO) continues to partner with leading institutions and experts to identify and classify emerging SARS-CoV-2 variants. These strains are classified as "variants of concern" (VOC) or "variants of interest" (VOI). According to WHO, VOCs are associated with increased transmissibility and/or virulence, a change in COVID-19 epidemiology or disease presentation or compromise the effectiveness of "public health and social measures or available diagnostics, vaccines, therapeutics." As of December 2021, 5 VOCs have been identified and include lineages B.1.1.7 (alpha), B.1.351 (beta), P.1 (gamma), B.1.617.2 (delta), and B.1.1.529 (omicron) all of which have been reported in the United States.[2,72,73] In early 2021, the FDA issued a letter to clinical laboratorians and health care providers warning that SARS-CoV-2 variants may not be detected by molecular tests, potentially resulting in false-negative results. Three EUA molecular tests—of which one was included in our review—were identified as potentially limited in their ability to detect variant strains.[74] According to the FDA letter, the S gene target of the TaqPath COVID-19 Combo Kit may have compromised sensitivity in the presence of the B.1.1.7 (alpha) variant, although both the FDA and Thermo Fisher Scientific, Inc., noted that the overall sensitivity of the test is unlikely to be impacted because of the inclusion of multiple targets.[74,75] Furthermore, the manufacturer theorizes that results suggesting S gene dropout (69–70del) may assist in the identification of samples infected with the alpha or omicron variant.[75–77] Of note is the BA.2 descendant lineage of omicron, which does not display the 69-70del and would therefore not be identified by dropout of the S gene.[78] In addition to mutations in the S gene, mutations in the N gene of the omicron variant may impact detection in molecular tests employing this target. The molecular tests included in our review were not among those identified by the FDA as expected to fail to detect SARS-CoV-2 omicron.[79] The inclusion of multiple gene targets is advantageous and may facilitate the identification of variant strains. The continued emergence of SARS-CoV-2 variants emphasizes the importance of assay design, and highlights the need for redundancy within the test, either by targeting multiple genes or at least 2 unique regions within the same gene.

It must also be noted that several features of COVID-19, such as the period of viral shedding and window of transmission, are not fully defined.[66] With this in mind, a key aspect to consider when assessing the clinical performance of molecular SARS-CoV-2 assays is whether a positive result indicates an active infection or simply the presence of viral RNA from a resolved infection. A study evaluating hospitalized patients with COVID-19 noted that throat swabs and sputum samples remained positive for 2 and 3 weeks, respectively, despite the resolution of COVID-19 symptoms.[80,81] Furthermore, replication-competent virus was not recovered from these patients beyond day 8 of symptoms, suggesting the period of active viral infection is likely shorter compared with detection of viral RNA.[80] In the future, the development of new assays that can help to discriminate active from past infections should be a focus for test manufacturers. This will be important to ensure proper allocation of limited resources, avoid unnecessary medical costs for patients, and only isolate patients for the period that they represent a risk for ongoing viral transmission.

Lastly, the frequency of false-negative molecular SARS-CoV-2 results requires further study. A study by Green and colleagues evaluated a large cohort of 27,377 SARS-CoV-2 molecular assays from 22,338 patients with testing performed by New York-Presbyterian laboratories and included a review of patients with repeat testing (n = 3432 patients [2413 initial negative results, 802 initial positive results]). Most testing was performed using the Roche SARS-CoV-2 test performed on the cobas 6800, with a smaller proportion performed using the ID NOW, Xpert Xpress, Panther Fusion, and in-house developed assays. In patients with repeat testing, 60 oscillated between positive and negative results, emphasizing the need for judicious interpretation of single-test laboratory results in the context of clinical symptoms.[66]

LIMITATIONS

This review is meant to provide an overview of the analytical and clinical performance of major commercial SARS-CoV-2 molecular assays in the United States. It is not intended to be an exhaustive summary of all available publications and relevant data. The observed analytical sensitivity (ie, LoD) data presented in **Table 3** were not always evaluated and published in the same units and/or using the same specimen type(s) as studies outlined in manufacturers' instructions for use, thereby limiting a direct comparison in many cases. In addition, information on observed analytical specificity (ie, cross-reactivity) was not available for several assays. Finally, the comparator assays used to determine clinical performance (ie, PPA/NPA) varied between studies, which further limits direct comparisons (see **Table 3**).

SUMMARY

Laboratory testing for SARS-CoV-2 has played a key role in the response to the COVID-19 pandemic. The rapid development of molecular assays has been crucial to identify positive cases, limit transmission of the virus, and manage patient care decisions. Overall, commercially available molecular assays for the detection of SARS-CoV-2 have demonstrated comparable performance. However, the sensitivity of these assays has been shown to vary, especially when performed at different time points during the course of COVID-19 disease and on different specimen types (eg, NP swabs vs oropharyngeal swabs). Although rapid, POC molecular tests may assist in making a timely diagnosis of COVID-19, a negative result may not definitively rule out the disease and follow-up testing using a laboratory-based assay may be required.[42,59,82,83] Future test development should focus on variant detection and discrimination, as well as differentiating active viral infection from persistent detection of viral RNA.

CLINICS CARE POINTS

- Greater than 200 SARS-CoV-2 molecular assays have received emergency use authorization by the U.S. Food and Drug Administration.
- In general, the analytic and clinical performance of commercially available molecular SARS-CoV-2 assays has been shown to be comparable by an independent evaluation of these methods.
- The selection of an appropriate commercial molecular SARS-CoV-2 assay is largely dependent on throughput, turnaround time, and cost considerations.
- The emergence of variant strains of SARS-CoV-2 may impact the performance characteristics of molecular assays, particularly those designed to target a single gene.
- Current SARS-CoV-2 molecular assays are unable to differentiate between active infection and persistent viral nucleic acid, which may lead to unnecessary isolation of non-infectious patients.

DISCLOSURE

M.J. Binnicker is a scientific advisory board member for DiaSorin Molecular and Mammoth Biosciences. M.R. Campbell has nothing to disclose.

REFERENCES

1. Coronavirus Resource Center. Johns Hopkins University & Medicine. Available at: https://coronavirus.jhu.edu/. Accessed December 21, 2021.
2. COVID Data Tracker. Centers for Disease Control and Prevention. Available at: https://covid.cdc.gov/covid-data-tracker/#variant-proportions. Accessed December 22, 2021.
3. In Vitro Diagnostics EUAs - Molecular Diagnostic Tests for SARS-CoV-2. U.S. Food & Drug Administration. Available at: https://www.fda.gov/medical-devices/coronavirus-disease-2019-covid-19-emergency-use-authorizations-medical-devices/in-vitro-diagnostics-euas-molecular-diagnostic-tests-sars-cov-2#individual-molecular. Accessed June 13, 2021.
4. SARS-CoV-2 Proficiency Testing and Quality Improvement Programs. College of American Pathologists. SARS-CoV-2 Proficiency Testing and Quality Improvement Programs. Accessed June 13, 2021.
5. COV2Q-A 2021 Participant Summary; Quality Cross Check-SARS-CoV-2, Molecular. College of American Pathologists; 2021.
6. Fung B, Gopez A, Servellita V, et al. Direct comparison of SARS-CoV-2 analytical limits of detection across seven molecular assays. J Clin Microbiol 2020;58(9): e01535-20.

7. Guidance for SARS-CoV-2 Point-of-Care and Rapid Testing. Centers for Disease Control and Prevention. 2021. Available at: https://www.cdc.gov/coronavirus/2019-ncov/lab/point-of-care-testing.html. Accessed June 13, 2021.

8. ID NOW™ COVID-19 Product Insert [package insert]. Scarborough (ME): Abbott Diagnostics Scarborough, Inc.; 2020.

9. Abbott RealTime SARS-CoV-2 [package insert]. Des Plaines (IL): Abbott Molecular, Inc.; 2020.

10. ID NOW COVID-19 [package insert]. Scarborough (ME): Abbott Diagnostics Scarborough, Inc.; 2020.

11. BD SARS-CoV-2 Reagents for BD MAXTM System [package insert]. Sparks (MD): Becton, Dickinson and Company; 2021.

12. BD BioGX SARS-CoV-2 Reagents for BD MAXTM System [package insert]. Sparks (MD): Becton, Dickinson and Company; 2020.

13. BioFire® COVID-19 Test Instructions for Use [package insert]. Salt Lake City (UT): BioFire Defense, LLC; 2020/2021.

14. Xpert® Omni SARS-CoV-2 Instructions for Use [package insert]. Sunnyvale (CA): Cepheid; 2021.

15. Xpert® Xpress SARS-CoV-2 Instructions for Use [package insert]. Sunnyvale (CA): Cepheid; 2021.

16. Simplexa™ COVID-19 Direct [package insert]. Cypress (CA): DiaSorin Molecular, LLC; 2021.

17. ePlex®SARS-CoV-2 Test Assay Manual [package insert]. Carlsbad (CA): GenMark Diagnostics, Inc.; 2020.

18. ARIES®SARS-CoV-2 Assay [package insert]. Austin (TX): Luminex Corporation; 2020.

19. Aptima® SARS-CoV-2 Assay (Panther® System) [package insert]. San Diego (CA): Hologic, Inc.; 2020.

20. SARS-CoV-2 Assay (Panther Fusion® System). [package insert]. San Diego (CA): Hologic, Inc.; 2020.

21. TaqPath™ COVID-19 Combo Kit Instructions for Use [package insert]. Pleasanton (CA): Life Technologies Corporation; 2020.

22. TaqPath™ COVID-19 Combo Kit. Thermo Fisher Scientific. Available at: https://www.thermofisher.com/order/catalog/product/A47814#/A47814. Accessed June 23, 2021.

23. TaqPath™ COVID-19 High Throughput Combo Kit. Thermo Fisher Scientific. Available at: https://www.thermofisher.com/order/catalog/product/A49869#/A49869. Accessed June 25, 2021.

24. ID NOW COVID-19 EUA letter of authorization. U.S. Food & Drug Administration. 2020. Available at: https://www.fda.gov/media/136522/download. Accessed June 23, 2021.

25. Abbott RealTime SARS-CoV-2 assay EUA letter of authorization. U.S. Food & Drug Administration. 2020. Available at: https://www.fda.gov/media/136255/download. Accessed June 23, 2021.

26. BioGX SARS-CoV-2 Reagents for BD MAX System EUA letter of authorization. U.S. Food & Drug Administration. 2020. Available at: https://www.fda.gov/media/136650/download. Accessed June 23, 2021.

27. BD SARS-CoV-2 Reagents for BD MAX System EUA letter of authorization. U.S. Food & Drug Administration. 2021. Available at: https://www.fda.gov/media/136813/download. Accessed June 23, 2021.

28. BioFire COVID-19 Test EUA letter of authorization. U.S. Food & Drug Administration. 2021. Available at: https://www.fda.gov/media/136356/download. Accessed June 23, 2021.
29. Xpert Omni SARS-CoV-2 EUA letter of authorization. U.S. Food & Drug Administration. 2021. Available at: https://www.fda.gov/media/144029/download. Accessed June 23, 2021.
30. Xpert Xpress SARS-CoV-2 EUA letter of authorization. U.S. Food & Drug Administration. 2021. Available at: https://www.fda.gov/media/136316/download. Accessed June 23, 2021.
31. ePlex SARS-CoV-2 Test EUA letter of authorization. U.S. Food & Drug Administration. 2020. Available at: https://www.fda.gov/media/136283/download. Accessed June 23, 2021.
32. Panther Fusion SARS-CoV-2 assay EUA letter of authorization. U.S. Food & Drug Administration. 2020. Available at: https://www.fda.gov/media/136153/download. Accessed June 23, 2021.
33. ARIES SARS-CoV-2 Assay EUA letter of authorization. U.S. Food & Drug Administration. 2020. Available at: https://www.fda.gov/media/136694/download. Accessed June 23, 2021.
34. Aptima SARS-CoV-2 assay EUA letter of authorization. U.S. Food & Drug Administration. 2021. Available at: https://www.fda.gov/media/138097/download. Accessed June 23, 2021.
35. TaqPath COVID-19 Combo Kit EUA letter of authorization. U.S. Food & Drug Administration. 2020. Available at: https://www.fda.gov/media/136113/download. Accessed June 23, 2021.
36. Cobas SARS-CoV-2 EUA letter of authorization. U.S. Food & Drug Administration. 2021. Available at: https://www.fda.gov/media/136046/download. Accessed June 23, 2021.
37. Amplitude Solution with TaqPath COVID-19 High-Throughput Combo Kit EUA letter of authorization. U.S. Food and Drug Administration. 2021. Available at: https://www.fda.gov/media/147535/download. Accessed June 25, 2021.
38. Molecular Diagnostic Template for Commercial Manufacturers. U.S. Food & Drug Administration. Published 2020. Accessed June 23, 2021.
39. cobas® SARS-CoV-2 [package insert]. Indianapolis (IN): Roche Diagnostics; 2021.
40. Amplitude™ Solution with the TaqPath™ COVID-19 High-Throughput Combo Kit Instructions for Use [package insert]. Pleasanton (CA): Thermo Fisher Scientific; 2021.
41. Lephart PR, Bachman MA, LeBar W, et al. Comparative study of four SARS-CoV-2 Nucleic Acid Amplification Test (NAAT) platforms demonstrates that ID NOW performance is impaired substantially by patient and specimen type. Diagn Microbiol Infect Dis 2021;99(1):115200.
42. Zhen W, Smith E, Manji R, et al. Clinical evaluation of three sample-to-answer platforms for detection of SARS-CoV-2. J Clin Microbiol 2020;58(8).
43. Degli-Angeli E, Dragavon J, Huang ML, et al. Validation and verification of the Abbott RealTime SARS-CoV-2 assay analytical and clinical performance. J Clin Virol 2020;129:104474.
44. Yanson K, Laviers W, Neely L, et al. Performance evaluation of the BD SARS-CoV-2 reagents for the BD MAX™ system. medRxiv 2021;59(12):e0101921.
45. Smith E, Zhen W, Manji R, et al. Analytical and clinical comparison of three nucleic acid amplification tests for SARS-CoV-2 Detection. J Clin Microbiol 2020;58(9).

46. Eckbo EJ, Locher K, Caza M, et al. Evaluation of the BioFire(R) COVID-19 test and Respiratory Panel 2.1 for rapid identification of SARS-CoV-2 in nasopharyngeal swab samples. Diagn Microbiol Infect Dis 2021;99(3):115260.

47. Loeffelholz MJ, Alland D, Butler-Wu SM, et al. Multicenter Evaluation of the Cepheid Xpert Xpress SARS-CoV-2 Test. *J Clin* Microbiol 2020;58(8):e00926-20.

48. Wolters F, van de Bovenkamp J, van den Bosch B, et al. Multi-center evaluation of cepheid xpert(R) xpress SARS-CoV-2 point-of-care test during the SARS-CoV-2 pandemic. J Clin Virol 2020;128:104426.

49. Zhen W, Manji R, Smith E, et al. Comparison of four molecular in vitro diagnostic assays for the detection of SARS-CoV-2 in nasopharyngeal specimens. J Clin Microbiol 2020;58(8).

50. Bordi L, Piralla A, Lalle E, et al. Rapid and sensitive detection of SARS-CoV-2 RNA using the Simplexa COVID-19 direct assay. J Clin Virol 2020;128:104416.

51. Uhteg K, Jarrett J, Richards M, et al. Comparing the analytical performance of three SARS-CoV-2 molecular diagnostic assays. J Clin Virol 2020;127:104384.

52. Pham J, Meyer S, Nguyen C, et al. Performance characteristics of a High-throughput automated transcription-mediated amplification test for SARS-CoV-2 Detection. J Clin Microbiol 2020;58(10):e01669-20.

53. Schneider M, Iftner T, Ganzenmueller T. Evaluation of the analytical performance and specificity of a SARS-CoV-2 transcription-mediated amplification assay. J Virol Methods 2021;294:114182.

54. Tanida K, Koste L, Koenig C, et al. Evaluation of the automated cartridge-based ARIES SARS-CoV-2 Assay (RUO) against automated Cepheid Xpert Xpress SARS-CoV-2 PCR as gold standard. Eur J Microbiol Immunol (Bp) 2020;10(3): 156–64.

55. Matsumura Y, Shimizu T, Noguchi T, et al. Comparison of 12 Molecular Detection Assays for Severe Acute Respiratory Syndrome Coronavirus 2 (SARS-CoV-2). J Mol Diagn 2021;23(2):164–70.

56. Abbott RealTime SARS-CoV-2 Instructions for Use [package insert]. Des Plaines (IL): Abbott Molecular, Inc.; 2020.

57. Cradic K, Lockhart M, Ozbolt P, et al. Clinical evaluation and utilization of multiple molecular in vitro diagnostic assays for the detection of SARS-CoV-2. Am J Clin Pathol 2020;154(2):201–7.

58. Dinnes J, Deeks JJ, Adriano A, et al. Rapid, point-of-care antigen and molecular-based tests for diagnosis of SARS-CoV-2 infection. Cochrane Database Syst Rev 2020;8:CD013705.

59. Mitchell SL, George KS. Evaluation of the COVID19 ID NOW EUA assay. J Clin Virol 2020;128:104429.

60. Rhoads DD, Cherian SS, Roman K, et al. Comparison of Abbott ID Now, DiaSorin Simplexa, and CDC FDA Emergency Use Authorization Methods for the Detection of SARS-CoV-2 from Nasopharyngeal and Nasal Swabs from Individuals Diagnosed with COVID-19. J Clin Microbiol 2020;58(8):e00760-20.

61. ABBOTT RELEASES ID NOW™ COVID-19 INTERIM CLINICAL STUDY RESULTS FROM 1,003 PEOPLE TO PROVIDE THE FACTS ON CLINICAL PERFORMANCE AND TO SUPPORT PUBLIC HEALTH. 2020. Abbott Available at: https://abbott.mediaroom.com/2020-10-07-Abbott-Releases-ID-NOW-TM-COVID-19-Interim-Clinical-Study-Results-from-1-003-People-to-Provide-the-Facts-on-Clinical-Performance-and-to-Support-Public-Health. Accessed June 23, 2021.

62. Lee CK, Tham JWM, Png S, et al. Clinical performance of Roche cobas 6800, Luminex ARIES, MiRXES Fortitude Kit 2.1, Altona RealStar, and applied Biosystems

TaqPath for SARS-CoV-2 detection in nasopharyngeal swabs. J Med Virol 2021; 93(7):4603–7.

63. ePlex®Respiratory Pathogen Panel 2 [package insert]. Carlsbad (CA): GenMark Diagnostics, Inc.; 2020.

64. Pujadas E, Ibeh N, Hernandez MM, et al. Comparison of SARS-CoV-2 detection from nasopharyngeal swab samples by the Roche cobas 6800 SARS-CoV-2 test and a laboratory-developed real-time RT-PCR test. J Med Virol 2020;92(9): 1695–8.

65. Lee J, Song JU. Diagnostic accuracy of the Cepheid Xpert Xpress and the Abbott ID NOW assay for rapid detection of SARS-CoV-2: a systematic review and meta-analysis. J Med Virol 2021;93(7):4523–31.

66. Green DA, Zucker J, Westblade LF, et al. Clinical performance of SARS-CoV-2 molecular tests. J Clin Microbiol 2020;58(8).

67. Younes N, Al-Sadeq DW, Al-Jighefee H, et al. Challenges in Laboratory Diagnosis of the Novel Coronavirus SARS-CoV-2. Viruses 2020;12(6):582.

68. Ai T, Yang Z, Hou H, et al. Correlation of Chest CT and RT-PCR Testing for Coronavirus Disease 2019 (COVID-19) in China: A Report of 1014 Cases. Radiology 2020;296(2):E32–40.

69. Song S, Wu F, Liu Y, et al. Correlation between chest CT findings and clinical features of 211 COVID-19 suspected patients in Wuhan, China. Open Forum Infect Dis 2020;7(6):ofaa171.

70. Xie X, Zhong Z, Zhao W, et al. Chest CT for Typical Coronavirus Disease 2019 (COVID-19) Pneumonia: Relationship to Negative RT-PCR Testing. Radiology 2020;296(2):E41–5.

71. He X, Lau EHY, Wu P, et al. Temporal dynamics in viral shedding and transmissibility of COVID-19. Nat Med 2020;26(5):672–5.

72. Tracking SARS-CoV-2 variants. World Health Organization. 2021. Available at: https://www.who.int/en/activities/tracking-SARS-CoV-2-variants/. Accessed December 22, 2021.

73. US COVID-19 Cases Caused by Variants. Centers for Disease Control and Prevention. 2021. Available at: https://www.cdc.gov/coronavirus/2019-ncov/variants/variant-cases.html. Accessed December 22, 2021.

74. Genetic Variants of SARS-CoV-2 May Lead to False Negative Results with Molecular Tests for Detection of SARS-CoV-2 - Letter to Clinical Laboratory Staff and Health Care Providers. U.S. Food & Drug Administration. Genetic Variants of SARS-CoV-2 May Lead to False Negative Results with Molecular Tests for Detection of SARS-CoV-2 - Letter to Clinical Laboratory Staff and Health Care Providers. 2021. Accessed June 22, 2021.

75. Emerging SARS-CoV-2 Mutations and Variants. Thermo Fisher Scientific. 2021. Available at: https://www.thermofisher.com/us/en/home/clinical/clinical-genomics/pathogen-detection-solutions/covid-19-sars-cov-2/mutations-variants.html. Accessed December 22, 2021.

76. Threat Assessment Brief. Rapid increase of a SARS-CoV-2 variant with multiple spike protein mutations observed in the United Kingdom. European Centre for Disease Prevention and Control. 2020. Available at: https://www.ecdc.europa.eu/en/publications-data/threat-assessment-brief-rapid-increase-sars-cov-2-variant-united-kingdom. Accessed June 22, 2021.

77. Peter Horby CH, Davies Nick, Edmunds John, et al. NERVTAG: presented to SAGE on 21/1/21. 2021. Available at: https://assets.publishing.service.gov.uk/government/uploads/system/uploads/attachment_data/file/961037/NERVTAG_note_on_B.1.1.7_severity_for_SAGE_77__1_.pdf. Accessed June 26, 2021.

78. Enhancing readiness for Omicron (B.1.1.529): Technical Brief and Priority Actions for Member States. World Health Organization; 2021.

79. SARS-CoV-2 Viral Mutations: Impact on COVID-19 Tests. U.S. Food & Drug Administration. 2021. Available at: https://www.fda.gov/medical-devices/coronavirus-covid-19-and-medical-devices/sars-cov-2-viral-mutations-impact-covid-19-tests#omicron-reduced. Accessed December 22, 2021.

80. Wolfel R, Corman VM, Guggemos W, et al. Virological assessment of hospitalized patients with COVID-2019. Nature 2020;581(7809):465–9.

81. Sethuraman N, Jeremiah SS, Ryo A. Interpreting diagnostic tests for SARS-CoV-2. JAMA 2020;323(22):2249–51.

82. Coronavirus (COVID-19) Update: FDA Informs Public About Possible Accuracy Concerns with Abbott ID NOW Point-of-Care Test. U.S. Food & Drug Administration. 2020. Available at: https://www.fda.gov/news-events/press-announcements/coronavirus-covid-19-update-fda-informs-public-about-possible-accuracy-concerns-abbott-id-now-point. Accessed July 17, 2021.

83. Thwe PM, Ren P. How many are we missing with ID NOW COVID-19 assay using direct nasopharyngeal swabs? Findings from a mid-sized academic hospital clinical microbiology laboratory. Diagn Microbiol Infect Dis 2020;98(2):115123.

84. Simplexa® COVID-19 Direct Kit. DiaSorin Molecular. Available at: https://molecular.diasorin.com/us/kit/simplexa-covid-19-direct-kit/. Accessed June 23, 2021.

The Successes and Challenges of SARS-CoV-2 Molecular Testing in the United States

Jennifer Dien Bard, PhD[a,b,*], N. Esther Babady, PhD[c,d]

KEYWORDS

- Challenges • COVID-19 • Molecular • SARS-CoV-2 • Successes

KEY POINTS

- Molecular technological advances throughout the SARS-CoV-2 pandemic are far superior to what was witnessed during the SARS pandemic.
- There have been many successes of SARS-CoV-2 molecular testing in the United States, including the development of rapid and novel molecular diagnostic assays; the leveraging of the high adaptability of molecular tests; and the integration of SARS-CoV-2 genotyping into public health, clinical, and research laboratories.
- The challenges related to SARS-CoV-2 molecular testing, such as regulatory hurdles, supply chain constraints, and laboratory preparation, should also be recognized and addressed to ensure that we are well prepared for future pandemics.

INTRODUCTION

On December 31, 2019, the world was alerted to the possibility of an emerging viral pathogen in Wuhan, China, causing a pneumonia syndrome reminiscent of the disease caused by the severe acute respiratory syndrome coronavirus (SARS-CoV). The first SARS pandemic, which similarly emerged in China, started in November 2002 and spread to 26 countries, causing 774 deaths over 11 months. SARS was defined in March 2003 after several months of investigation, and the whole genome of SARS-CoV was available approximately 1 month later.[1] As such, the majority of SARS diagnoses made over the duration of the pandemic were primarily based on

[a] Department of Pathology and Laboratory Medicine, Children's Hospital Los Angeles, 4650 Sunset Blvd, MS#32, Los Angeles, CA 90027, USA; [b] Department of Pathology, Keck School of Medicine of the University of Southern California, Los Angeles, CA, USA; [c] Clinical Microbiology Service, Department of Pathology and Laboratory Medicine, Memorial Sloan Kettering Cancer Center, 327 East 64th Street, CLM-522, NY 10065, USA; [d] Infectious Disease Service, Department of Medicine, Memorial Sloan Kettering Cancer Center, New York, NY, USA
* Corresponding author. Department of Pathology and Laboratory Medicine, Children's Hospital Los Angeles, 4650 Sunset Blvd, MS#32, Los Angeles, CA 90027, USA
E-mail address: jdienbard@chla.usc.edu

Clin Lab Med 42 (2022) 147–160
https://doi.org/10.1016/j.cll.2022.02.007
0272-2712/22/© 2022 Elsevier Inc. All rights reserved.
labmed.theclinics.com

the clinical case definition established by the World Health Organization (WHO), which had a sensitivity of 26% and specificity of 96%.[2] Fast forward 17 years and scientists in China reported the identification of a novel coronavirus, eventually called SARS-CoV-2, on January 9, 2020, as the cause of the coronavirus disease 2019 (COVID-19) syndrome. The identification of SARS-CoV-2 was less than 2 weeks from the initial report made to the WHO, and the whole genome of the virus was made publicly available the next day on January 10, 2020. By January 13, 2020, the first protocol for a reverse-transcriptase polymerase chain reaction (RT-PCR) for laboratory diagnosis was published.[3] The incredible speed with which SARS-CoV-2 was identified and diagnostic methods developed was due in great part to the wider use of molecular methods in 2019 compared with 2002 during the SARS pandemic. From rapid, point-of-care RT-PCR tests to next-generation sequencing (NGS) assays, molecular methods have played a critical role in this pandemic. The goal of this review is to highlight the successes of molecular testing in the United States over the course of the pandemic and to also discuss the many challenges encountered and how the lessons learned during this pandemic, which is ongoing as of the time of writing, should allow for improved preparation of the next.

SUCCESSES
Rapid Development of Molecular Tests

The initial discovery and identification of SARS-CoV-2 as a novel virus relied heavily on the use of molecular diagnostic assays[4]. In their study, Zhu and colleagues used a commercial multiplexed respiratory viral panel (RespiFinderSmart22kit, PathoFinder BV) that targeted 18 viruses and 4 bacteria. The lack of detection on the multiplexed panel prompted further investigations of the underlying cause of this pneumonia syndrome using unbiased whole-genome sequencing on both clinical samples and viruses grown in human respiratory epithelial cell cultures. The assembled genomes closely matched those of known beta coronaviruses, allowing development of a targeted, pan-beta coronavirus real-time PCR that further confirmed the presence of this novel virus in clinical samples. This initial study foreshadowed the vital role that molecular diagnostic methods would have in the management of this disease.

The rapid availability of the first SARS-CoV-2 genomes, which were sequenced and deposited in the China National Microbiological Data Center in early January, was crucial for laboratories across the world to start designing primers and probes to detect unique viral genome regions of this novel virus.[5] In the United States, the first published RT-PCR assay was designed by the Centers for Disease Control and Prevention (CDC) and used to confirm the first case of COVID-19 from a returning traveler from Wuhan, China.[6] This assay initially targeted three distinct sequences of the gene encoding the nucleocapsid (N) protein of SARS-CoV-2, with a positive result requiring the detection of at least 2 of the 3 targets.[7] On February 4, the CDC became the first institution to receive emergency use authorization (EUA) only regulatory status from the US Food and Drug Administration (FDA) for their COVID-19 RT-PCR. Initial rollout of the CDC tests to public health laboratories was met with several challenges secondary to inconsistent assay performance, which required the test to be modified and optimized to focus on the detection of 2 instead of 3 sequences of the N gene, with results reported either positive (two targets detected) or presumptive (only one target detected). Results were invalid if the internal control, human RNAse P, was not detected.[8] Despite the delays in the rollout of the CDC assay, the publicly available information on the primers and probes of the CDC COVID-19 test offered many high-complexity laboratories in the United States the option to adopt or modify the CDC test to support case ascertainment of COVID-19 at the local level. In the early days of the pandemic in the United States, this was a major success of molecular method. The CDC COVID-19 test was eventually removed from the list of FDA EUA tests in the summer of 2021, at a point when other commercial assays had become readily available.

Development of Novel Molecular Tests

In addition to well-established nucleic acid amplification tests (NAATs), emerging molecular technologies including clustered regularly interspaced short palindromic repeats (CRISPR)-based detection[9] and digital PCRs were approved for in vitro diagnostic (IVD) use. Before the pandemic, CRISPR-based assays for infectious diseases were just beginning to show promise for use as a point-of-care diagnostic tool for Zika viruses and dengue viruses.[10,11] During the pandemic, 2 assays, the Sherlock CRISPR SARS-CoV-2 test (Sherlock Biosciences, Inc) and the SARS-CoV-2 DETECTR (Mammoth Biosciences, Inc.) received FDA EUA status for SARS-CoV-2 detection. Both methods used a combination of reverse transcriptase-loop-mediated isothermal amplification (RT-LAMP) and CRISPR-based detection of the target RNA sequences. Although ultimately the goal of these CRISPR-based methods is detection at the point of care, the current EUA assays still require instruments to measure fluorescence (e.g., ABI 7500 Dx platforms or BioTek Plater reader). Unlike CRISPR-based methods, digital droplet PCR (ddPCR) has been in use for several years in the research space but had yet to achieve IVD status for the diagnosis of any infectious disease[12]. Two assays, the Bio-Rad SARS-CoV-2 ddPCR test (Bio-Rad Laboratories, Inc.) and FastPlex Triplex SARS-CoV-2 (PreciGenome LLC) have now received FDA EUA status. Although there are currently no peer-reviewed publications on these specific assays, several studies have reported increased sensitivity of ddPCR assays compared with quantitative PCR (qPCR), showing its potential as a valid alternative.[13,14] Furthermore, the ability of ddPCR to provide absolute quantification could fill an existing gap related to the inability to perform viral load measurement for disease monitoring and infection control purposes. For the time being, currently authorized ddPCR platforms remain qualitative only and turnaround time to results are longer than for most qPCR instruments. Digital PCR instruments are also not as widely available in clinical microbiology laboratories as PCR thermocyclers.

One of the major successes of molecular testing during the pandemic, was the availability of rapid, point-of-care molecular tests. The ID Now COVID-19 test (Abbott Diagnostics Inc., Scarborough, ME) is an isothermal NAAT designed for testing on the ID Now platform, which is cleared for use at the point of care and provides results in as little as 5 minutes. Early studies comparing the performance of the ID Now COVID-19 test to other PCR tests showed sensitivity ranging from 55% to 98% when compared with SARS-CoV-2 PCRs, highlighting the lower sensitivity of RT-LAMP methods compared with PCR.[15–18] The pandemic also gave rise to the first-ever FDA EUAs conferred for Clinical Laboratory Improvement Amendment (CLIA)-waived IVD molecular assays that can be performed at home. These assays combine the speed of antigen testing with the sensitivity expected from conventional laboratory molecular tests.[19] Four platforms, the Lucira COVID-19 All-in-One test, the Lucira CHECK-IT COVID-19 test, the Cue COVID-19 test, and the Detect COVID-19 test are currently on the market. All 4 tests use RT-LAMP to amplify and detect SARS-CoV-2 RNA in less than 30 minutes from self-collected nasal swabs. Whereas these assays provide an opportunity for individuals to self-test at home, they are still not readily available and are relatively expensive compared with rapid antigen tests. There are also currently no available peer-reviewed data on their clinical and analytical performance compared with real-time RT-PCR tests, but given that amplification is isothermal, it is expected that sensitivity would be lower (though higher than for rapid antigen tests). Data from the manufacturer report the limit of detection (LOD) as 800 to 1300 copies/mL. Therefore, a negative test in a symptomatic patient should be confirmed with a PCR test, which is similar to algorithms that rely on antigen testing.

High Adaptability of Molecular Testing

Not only was molecular testing critical for diagnosing symptomatic individuals with COVID-19, it played a key role in keeping places such as health care settings and schools as safe as possible through surveillance testing of asymptomatic individuals. The ability to maintain highly sensitive and accurate testing at a large scale was largely due to the inherent adaptability of molecular testing. The ability to modify nearly any aspect of the preanalytical and analytical components of a PCR testing protocol, from collection devices to amplification techniques, allows it to be tailored to the specific needs of the setting in which it is deployed while optimizing its robustness to shortages in supplies and labor.

Preanalytical accommodations

Alternate Sample Collection Devices. Shortages of collection devices, such as swabs, prompted commercial companies and laboratories to pursue alternative methods for specimen collection. A lack of viral transport media (VTM) prompted the exploration of VTM-free protocols, such as collection in phosphate-buffered saline (PBS), Hanks' balanced salt solution (HBSS) or use of "dry" swabs that would be eluted in a small amount of media upon arrival at the testing laboratory. The performance of PCR in the detection of SARS-CoV-2 from these alternate buffers have been demonstrated to be comparable to VTM.[20,21] Detection of SARS-CoV-2 RNA by PCR appears to be robust at various temperatures and after exposure to multiple freeze thaw cycles. The logarithmic increase in testing needs early in the pandemic resulted in a sudden and dramatic shortage in swabs that was mitigated either by the foresight to hoard tens of thousands of swabs for internal use, the acquisition of swabs from less well-known sources, or to explore the use of 3D-printed swabs. The rapid adoption of 3D printing is a prime example of the creativity and the perseverance of laboratorians to dodge interruptions in clinical service. The performance of these swabs was found to be equivalent to flocked swabs, paving the way for a stable supply of this critical resource.[22]

Alternative Sample Types. Molecular testing is technically agnostic to sample type. However, in order for results to be meaningful for a provider, the body site must be considered clinically relevant and the sample type must have undergone sufficient validation. Although the collection of nasopharyngeal swabs (NPS) is considered the gold standard specimen collection method for SARS-CoV-2, several challenges have prompted commercial partners and CLIA-certified laboratories to explore alternate specimen sources that does not require specialized collection devices (e.g., NPSs and VTM). These challenges include the often painful or uncomfortable collection process, the need for personal protective equipment (PPE) for health care workers performing testing and, as mentioned above, supply chain shortages.[23] Thus, considerable efforts were made to explore and implement alternate clinical specimen types for the molecular detection of SARS-CoV-2. Currently, the Infectious Diseases Society of America (IDSA) and the Centers for Disease Control and Prevention (CDC) have approved other specimen types for SARS-CoV-2 testing including oropharyngeal swabs (OPS), midturbinate swabs (MTS), anterior nares swabs (ANS), saliva, and lower respiratory specimens. Other biological specimens including stool, blood,

CSF, and urine have also been explored with limited success.[23] Saliva samples, which had not routinely been used to diagnose respiratory tract infections before the pandemic, became central to community testing programs in schools and universities. Much attention has been given to saliva because of the ease of collection, and the lack of need for a swab, buffer solution, and even PPE.[24] The sensitivity of molecular tests on saliva samples varied widely depending on the assays but performance as high as 95% has been reported,[24–26] when compared with PCR testing on nasopharyngeal swabs and several assays have received FDA EUA for detection of SARS-CoV-2.[19] As data emerged on the utility of alternative samples for SARS-CoV-2 detection, saliva samples as well as nasal and MTS samples were preferred over the use of the more established OPS[27]. The success of molecular testing on saliva and other non-nasopharyngeal sample types will likely have a major impact on the diagnosis and management of many other infectious diseases post this pandemic.

Analytical Accommodations

Molecular testing approaches for SARS-CoV-2 have the flexibility to improve the speed and throughput of testing by bypassing external extraction steps and through specimen pooling algorithms, respectively. Neither approach is considered novel and they have been an integral part of laboratory medicine for many years before the COVID-19 pandemic. For example, many multiplexed syndromic testing panels for respiratory infections and gastroenteritis are built as sample-to-answer instruments that integrate nucleic acid extraction with amplification and signal detection. Results are typically available within 1 h.[28] The ability to modify or eliminate steps is an important feature of any molecular test, and particularly for PCR-based testing, as it can significantly reduce the time to result without affecting analytical sensitivity.[18,29]

With regard to specimen pooling, combining multiple specimens before nucleic acid extraction can be easily accommodated from the analytical perspective as the extraction process itself remains the same. Specimen pooling algorithms have been successfully deployed for other infectious diseases such as HIV,[30] with minimal effects on sensitivity. Pooling studies for SARS-CoV-2 using PCR-based methods and other molecular approaches like CRISPR have found that sensitivity can be maintained when up to 5 specimens are pooled, with decreases thereafter as the number of specimens included in the pool increases.[31] Pooling can be an effective approach for asymptomatic surveillance in the community to facilitate early detection of COVID-19, provided that disease prevalence remains low.[32]

Application of Molecular Testing for SARS-CoV-2 Genomic Surveillance

The availability of NGS to investigate the initial Wuhan clusters and produce the first complete genome of SARS-CoV-2 within days was crucial to diagnostic assay development and to the molecular characterization of this novel virus.[4] As a public health tool, NGS has had a transformative role in replacing older typing methods to investigate outbreaks and for surveillance of known and emerging pathogens.[33–35] Genomic surveillance of SARS-CoV-2 by NGS is without a doubt one of the biggest successes of molecular testing during the pandemic and highlights the benefits of global collaboration and open data sharing.

The initial investment in whole genome sequencing of SARS-CoV-2 was made by research and public health laboratories interested in monitoring and investigating SARS-CoV-2 genome evolution.[36] However, when genomic changes, including single nucleotide polymorphisms (SNPs) and deletions, were observed to impact the virus transmission, infectivity and detection by diagnostic tests, the interest and need for genomic surveillance expanded significantly.[37,38] In November 2020, Public Health

England reported an increased in COVID-19 cases associated a variant of SARS-CoV-2, now referred to as the Alpha variant, that was characterized by key changes (N501Y and P618H) and deletions (del69–70) in the spike gene[39]. These changes affected the performance of assays targeting the S gene and were easily identified as S gene target failures (SGTFs) when using the affected PCR tests. The impact of emerging mutations in the SARS-CoV-2 genome over the course of the pandemic underscored the importance of the approach taken early in the pandemic to design molecular tests with multiple genomic targets. With the continual accrual of global data on the impact of emerging variants on the analytical performance of molecular diagnostic tests, the FDA issued guidance for all manufacturers of SARS-CoV-2 diagnostics tests to monitor and confirmed continued performance of their EUA tests.[40] The approval of SARS-CoV-2 vaccines in the fall of 2020 provided further incentive to use NGS to monitor genome evolution and the potential for emerging variants to reduce neutralization from antibodies acquired through natural infection, vaccination, or through monoclonal antibody therapeutics.

As genomic surveillance of SARS-CoV-2 expanded, the WHO in collaboration with other public health networks including the US SARS-CoV-2 Interagency Group (SIG), developed a naming scheme to classify variants based on their potential impact on the pandemic, including variants of interest (VOI) and variants of concerns (VOC). SARS-CoV-2 variants with mutations that are predicted or known to affect transmissibility, disease severity, immunity, diagnostic accuracy, or therapeutic success were considered VOIs. VOCs were VOIs for which there was actual evidence of increased transmissibility or increased virulence, decreased protection from vaccination or previous infection, diagnostic failures or reduced effectiveness of therapeutics.[41,42] As VOIs and VOCs started to emerge in many countries, a naming scheme that used the Greek alphabet was developed by WHO experts to facilitate discussions by nonscientific audiences and to prevent the stigma associated with naming VOIs/VOCs after the countries in which they were first identified. Beyond global surveillance testing to monitor emerging SARS-CoV-2 lineages, NGS performed in clinical laboratories provided data that supported local hospital outbreak investigations and transmission events or local efforts to monitor and establish links between emerging variants and vaccines breakthroughs.[43–46]

Implementation of NGS in clinical laboratories for genomic surveillance was challenging, particularly as traditional NAAT-based diagnostic testing required constant human, material, and financial support throughout the pandemic. Furthermore, for most clinical virology and microbiology laboratories, NGS was not a technique used routinely and thus to perform surveillance in-house required a significant amount of new investment not only in NGS instrumentation but also in technologists with strong skillsets for molecular techniques as well as in staff with the ability to use bioinformatic tools for data analysis of SARS-CoV-2 sequences. The complexity of NGS for routine surveillance of SARS-CoV-2 prompted the development of targeted PCR to identify specific VOC/VOI through detection of known key mutations[47,48]. This approach took advantages of existing skills and infrastructures in clinical laboratories to rapidly identify VOC/VOI. However, as successive waves of the pandemic increased and decreased and the frequencies of VOC/VOI changed frequently, the utility of targeted approaches became limited.

NGS has become the method of choice for surveillance of SARS-CoV-2 as it is agnostic to variants. However, the use of NGS comes with its own set of challenges that include the introduction of artifacts into output datasets by the methods (tiled amplicons vs metagenomics), and platforms (e.g., long reads vs short reads) used. It is essential that the chosen bioinformatic pipelines are validated to reduce the risk of bias in data interpretation and standardization[49]. Despite the increased complexity of NGS, there is increasing interest and a potential role in offering SARS-CoV-2 genotyping as a clinical test as it may contribute to the selection or avoidance of some monoclonal antibody or antiviral therapies.[50]

The success of NGS during the SARS-CoV-2 pandemic was also due in part to the increase in data sharing globally, primarily through the Global Initiative on Sharing All Influenza Data (GISAID) initiative, which pivoted early in the pandemic to developing and providing tools that enabled validation and free data sharing of SARS-CoV-2 genomes as well as for visualization and real-time tracking.[51] As of February 2022, more than 7,700,000 SARS-CoV-2 genomes have been submitted to GISAID. Although submissions are heavily biased toward laboratories from high and middle-income countries, the free access and the extent of sharing of genomic data have been unprecedented and has allowed for truly global surveillance of viral evolution. In addition to GISAID and other data repository tools (e.g., NCBI GenBank), open software platforms such as Nextstrain and Phylogenetic Assignment of Named Global Outbreak Lineages (PANGOLIN) have facilitated the assignments of SARS-CoV-2 lineages, particularly for laboratories with limited bioinformatics skills.[52–55]

CHALLENGES AND TRIALS

Although the successes of molecular testing are worthy of celebration, we would be remiss to not discuss their failures as well. Among them are the bureaucratic failures that severely delayed the deployment of these vital tests at a critical moment early in the pandemic, global supply chain bottlenecks, the inability of molecular tests to assess contagiousness, the paucity of skilled laboratory scientists to meet testing demands, and the lack of coordination with state and federal public health laboratories.

US FDA Regulatory Hurdles

Although the CDC was able to achieve EUA status for their COVID-19 assay, most clinical laboratories were not equipped to undertake the challenges associated with the complexity and length of an FDA EUA submission. However, as cases of COVID-19 started to increase and local transmission became evident, clinical laboratories and commercial entities appropriately worked diligently to submit SARS-CoV-2 PCR tests for FDA review and approval. It became immediately apparent that a significant challenge was the lack of a readily available gold standard. Most laboratories at the beginning of the pandemic did not have access to samples positive for SARS-CoV-2 or to well-characterized viral isolates. Furthermore, guidance was issued early in 2020 advising against the performance of viral cultures on any respiratory samples, unless done in a Biosafety level 3 (BSL-3) laboratory, which is not available in many clinical laboratories. These hurdles made establishing the performance characteristics of an assay for this novel pathogen quite challenging. Ultimately, on February 28, the FDA issued a guidance for high-complexity laboratories and diagnostic manufacturers that provided a simplified path to developing and obtaining EUA clearance for molecular diagnostic tests.[56] This guidance allowed laboratories to perform validation using viral RNA transcripts in the absence of true clinical samples. Only after that point were both clinical laboratories and commercial vendors able to move forward with developing molecular tests for SARS-CoV-2 RNA detection. In a matter of a few months, hundreds of SARS-CoV-2 molecular tests became available.

The Supply Chain

One of the biggest challenges of the pandemic has undoubtedly been an inadequate supply chain. Global travel and economic output came to a standstill in spring 2020 because of the strict lockdowns occurring in many parts of the world simultaneously. At the same time, once molecular tests were implemented in clinical laboratories, cases surged and with it, an unexpected and unprecedented demand for rapid testing. This led to a significant mismatch between supplies and demand for one of the most critical operations during the pandemic. The challenges associated with limited supplies from sample collection devices (e.g., viral transport media, nasopharyngeal swabs) to PCR reagents and instruments, created the need for validating alternative molecular testing methods including RT-LAMP and transcription-mediated amplification (TMA), and alternative sample types to minimize the need for specialized collection kits or NAAT reagents. The first nonPCR NAATs to become commercially available were based on isothermal amplification (e.g., ID Now COVID-19 Test, Abbott Inc.; Solana SARS-CoV-2 Assay, Quidel Inc.), with some having the added benefit of being able to use dry nasal swabs.[19] As described previously, the analytical sensitivity of various RT-LAMP assays was lower than PCR. However, the performance of SARS-CoV-2 TMA assays (e.g., Aptima SARS-CoV-2 Assay, Hologic Inc.) showed similar sensitivity and specificity compared with PCRs, allowing for further expansion of sensitive and accurate molecular tests during the pandemic.[57]

The challenges associated with the supply chain and the costs of molecular tests led to increasing delays in resulting turn-around times early in the pandemic. In response, nonmolecular tests, primarily antigen-based, were developed to further expand testing and also fill the gap for rapid, point-of-care testing. To date, over 25 antigen tests have received the FDA EUA status.[58] The lower sensitivity of antigen assays, which do not employ amplification methods, compared with molecular tests, was an anticipated challenge based on prior experience with rapid influenza diagnostics tests (RIDTs). Numerous studies have now shown rapid antigen tests for SARS-CoV-2 to have sensitivities as low as 35% in asymptomatic patients compared with PCRs, though this improves to over 90% for samples with high viral loads (e.g., Ct values < 30).[59–62] Results of studies varied widely depending on the patient population tested (e.g., symptomatic vs asymptomatic patients), the type of tests (e.g., lateral-flow assays vs high-throughput chemiluminescence assays) and the timing of testing (e.g., early vs late infection). As such, recommendations from the IDSA guidelines still support the use of molecular over antigen testing whenever possible.[63] The CDC guidelines similarly suggest an approach that takes into consideration the patient population and the goal of testing to optimize the use of antigen testing with recommendations to follow up negative antigen tests with molecular testing in cases of high suspicion of infection.[64]

Dead or Alive?

A major challenge for all types of diagnostic testing for SARS-CoV-2 is the inability to discriminate between actively replicating virus and viral RNA fragments. This is particularly the case for highly sensitive molecular testing assays. Early in the pandemic, the CDC recommended performing a NAAT test for "clearance" of infection. However, it became rapidly evident that it was not uncommon to detect viral RNA fragments for weeks or months after an individual has completely recovered from COVID-19.[65] As such, the CDC modified their previous guidance to remove testing for clearance and shift to a time-based strategy for safely returning back to work or society.[66]

Some have championed the use of viral cultures to determine active infection or "infectivity,"[67] which is unrealistic in practice as performing viral cultures is a time consuming process that requires the availability of a BSL-3 laboratory. Due to low sensitivity, viral cultures are also considered a suboptimal reference method compared with NAAT and the reason for why the majority of clinical laboratories have abandoned its use for the detection of most viral pathogens.[68]

The use of rapid antigen tests (RAT) has also been proposed as a scalable and relatively cheap means to detect "infectious" cases. The association between a positive antigen test and contagiousness has been attributed to its lower sensitivity—meaning it should in theory only detect samples with high viral load or low cycle threshold (Ct) values seen by PCR.[69] Unfortunately, data correlating Ct values and infectivity are lacking and the widespread use of RAT has its own unique challenges. Additional discussion on the strengths and weaknesses of RAT for SARS-CoV-2 is covered in a separate article in this issue.

Lastly, a molecular approach that has been proposed to identify actively replicating virus compared with "dead" virus is the detection of minus-strand SARS-CoV-2 RNA[70] or subgenomic RNA.[71] These molecular testing approaches are tools that may assist in the determination of infectiousness in certain clinical contexts, such as in immunocompromised patients with prolonged shedding,[72] and could inform isolation strategies in a hospital setting.[70] However, conflicting data have been reported for the role of subgenomic RNA as a suitable indicator of actively replicating virus.[73] Clinical laboratories that wish to explore either minus-strand SARS-CoV RNA or subgenomic RNA RT-PCR should do so in the context of clinical and epidemiologic findings.

Limited Molecular Testing Capability and Shortage of Highly Skilled Molecular Technologists

The lack of molecular testing capability in many clinical laboratories, particularly nonacademic medical centers, was and remains a significant challenge. Early in the pandemic the only tests available had to be performed in laboratory spaces approved for high complexity testing. Unfortunately, many clinical laboratories lack that level of infrastructure and expertise. This shifted the testing demand to reference laboratories, which quickly became overwhelmed themselves. It was not uncommon to hear about testing delays of up to 10 days from time of collection. As commercial kits were granted EUA by the FDA, the dependency on reference laboratories shifted to dependency on diagnostic companies that offer moderately complexed testing kits (i.e., sample-to-answer molecular tests) that do not require external extraction step and molecular expertise.

The availability of rapid, point-of-care and at-home testing also highlighted one of the major challenges of the pandemic, namely the staffing of high-complexity laboratories with skilled technologists to run molecular testing. The shortage of qualified staff preceded the pandemic but the problem was greatly exacerbated by the stresses placed upon the laboratory by the massive testing demand. Many clinical laboratories resorted to collaboration with their research counterparts to find the necessary people with appropriate skills for performing molecular clinical testing. This also required that licensing be suspended in many places for the duration of the pandemic. While the COVID-19 pandemic is still ongoing, efforts to anticipate futures challenges will need to consider how solutions implemented during this pandemic to manage staffing and supply shortages can be readily reactivated when the next pandemic hits.

In order to learn from this challenge, steps must be put in place before the next pandemic. These include significant investments in clinical laboratories including (1) establishment of molecular testing infrastructure in clinical laboratories; (2) increase in the training of medical laboratory scientists with a focus on development of molecular skills; and (3) requirement of doctoral level trained clinical microbiologists to oversee clinical microbiology laboratories. Unless improvements are made it is very likely that the laboratory community will encounter the same issues as with the COVID-19 pandemic. An opinion editorial in the New York Times by Dr. Robin Patel (Mayo Clinic) and Dr. Stefano Bertuzzi (CEO, America Society for Microbiology) suggested the need for a "biomedical scientists version of the national guard" that would be activated in times of need to prevent the staffing challenges experienced during the COVID-19 pandemic.[64]

Clinical Versus Public Health Laboratories

The dependency of SARS-CoV-2 molecular testing, particularly early on in the pandemic, brought to light the disconnect between clinical laboratories and their public health laboratory partners. As per the WHO, a strong national infectious disease diagnostic and surveillance testing strategy should have a robust public health laboratory network as well as clinical laboratories and emphasizes the importance of the interconnectedness of both.[74] For clinical laboratories, collaboration with public health laboratories is critical as it may be the only source for clinical specimens required for validation of molecular testing platforms. In hindsight, the lack of standardized assistance and services offered to clinical laboratories in the US may have contributed to delays in implementation of SARS-CoV-2 molecular testing in laboratories capable of performing high complexity testing.

Early recognition of the critical role of the clinical laboratories in combating a pandemic is needed. An approach akin to the Laboratory Response Network for detection of biological terrorism that includes clinical laboratories as sentinel laboratories for early detection of the pathogen of interests may be considered. Standardization from the CDC level to all public health laboratories regardless of states or regions to offer early support to clinical laboratories can also help mitigate some of the issues encountered during this pandemic. This would include providing specimens or standards to accelerate the validation and implementation of the molecular test. The COVID-19 pandemic has taught us that there is no success in being siloed.

SUMMARY

Since the start of the pandemic, we continue to witness significant innovation in the laboratory and at the point of care. The pandemic also expedited the advancement of infectious diseases genomic surveillance in both public health and clinical laboratories for variant detection and outbreak investigation. As such, molecular development has grown by leaps and bounds over the past 2 years and it behooves us to (i) take advantage of this innovation wave and explore opportunities for other infectious diseases and (ii) recognize and learn from the challenges encountered to ensure that we are not victims to it when the next pandemic arrives on our shores.

REFERENCES

1. Peiris JS, Yuen KY, Osterhaus AD, et al. The severe acute respiratory syndrome. N Engl J Med 2003;349:2431–41.
2. Rainer TH, Cameron PA, Smit D, et al. Evaluation of WHO criteria for identifying patients with severe acute respiratory syndrome out of hospital: prospective observational study. BMJ 2003;326:1354–8.
3. Available at: https://www.who.int/emergencies/diseases/novel-coronavirus-2019/interactive-timeline#event-18. Accessed December 15, 2021.
4. Zhu N, Zhang D, Wang W, et al. A novel coronavirus from patients with pneumonia in China, 2019. N Engl J Med 2020;382:727–33.
5. Lu R, Zhao X, Li J, et al. Genomic characterisation and epidemiology of 2019 novel coronavirus: implications for virus origins and receptor binding. Lancet 2020;395:565–74.

6. Holshue ML, DeBolt C, Lindquist S, et al, Washington State -nCo VCIT. First case of 2019 novel coronavirus in the United States. N Engl J Med 2020;382:929–36.
7. Available at: https://www.cdc.gov/coronavirus/2019-ncov/downloads/rt-pcr-panel-primer-probes.pdf. Accessed December 15, 2021.
8. Available at: https://www.fda.gov/media/134922/download. Accessed December 15, 2021.
9. Ganbaatar U, Liu C. CRISPR-based COVID-19 testing: toward next-generation point-of-care diagnostics. Front Cell Infect Microbiol 2021;11:663949.
10. Gootenberg JS, Abudayyeh OO, Kellner MJ, et al. Multiplexed and portable nucleic acid detection platform with Cas13, Cas12a, and Csm6. Science 2018;360:439–44.
11. Gootenberg JS, Abudayyeh OO, Lee JW, et al. Nucleic acid detection with CRISPR-Cas13a/C2c2. Science 2017;356:438–42.
12. Available at: https://www.sciencedirect.com/science/article/abs/pii/S0196439918300114?via%3Dihub. Accessed December 15, 2021.
13. Alteri C, Cento V, Antonello M, et al. Detection and quantification of SARS-CoV-2 by droplet digital PCR in real-time PCR negative nasopharyngeal swabs from suspected COVID-19 patients. PLoS One 2020;15:e0236311.
14. Suo T, Liu X, Feng J, et al. ddPCR: a more accurate tool for SARS-CoV-2 detection in low viral load specimens. Emerg Microbes Infect 2020;9:1259–68.
15. Basu A, Zinger T, Inglima K, et al. Performance of abbott ID now COVID-19 rapid nucleic acid amplification test using nasopharyngeal swabs transported in viral transport media and dry nasal swabs in a New York city academic institution. J Clin Microbiol 2020;58(8):e01136-20.
16. Harrington A, Cox B, Snowdon J, et al. Comparison of abbott id now and abbott m2000 methods for the detection of SARS-CoV-2 from nasopharyngeal and nasal swabs from symptomatic patients. J Clin Microbiol 2020;58(8):e00798-20.
17. Rhoads DD, Cherian SS, Roman K, et al. Comparison of abbott id now, diasorin simplexa, and CDC FDA emergency use authorization methods for the detection of SARS-CoV-2 from Nasopharyngeal and Nasal Swabs from Individuals Diagnosed with COVID-19. J Clin Microbiol 2020;58(8):e00760-20.
18. Smithgall MC, Scherberkova I, Whittier S, et al. Comparison of cepheid xpert xpress and abbott ID now to roche cobas for the rapid detection of SARS-CoV-2. J Clin Virol 2020;128:104428.
19. Available at: https://www.fda.gov/medical-devices/coronavirus-disease-2019-covid-19-emergency-use-authorizations-medical-devices/in-vitro-diagnostics-euas-molecular-diagnostic-tests-sars-cov-2#imft3. Accessed December 15, 2021.
20. Padgett LR, Kennington LA, Ahls CL, et al. Polyester nasal swabs collected in a dry tube are a robust and inexpensive, minimal self-collection kit for SARS-CoV-2 testing. PLoS One 2021;16:e0245423.
21. Perchetti GA, Nalla AK, Huang ML, et al. Validation of SARS-CoV-2 detection across multiple specimen types. J Clin Virol 2020;128:104438.
22. Decker SJ, Goldstein TA, Ford JM, et al. 3-Dimensional printed alternative to the standard synthetic flocked nasopharyngeal swabs used for coronavirus disease 2019 testing. Clin Infect Dis 2021;73:e3027–32.
23. Wang W, Xu Y, Gao R, et al. Detection of SARS-CoV-2 in different types of clinical specimens. JAMA 2020;323:1843–4.
24. Wyllie AL, Fournier J, Casanovas-Massana A, et al. Saliva or nasopharyngeal swab specimens for detection of SARS-CoV-2. N Engl J Med 2020;383:1283–6.

25. Babady NE, McMillen T, Jani K, et al. Performance of severe acute respiratory syndrome coronavirus 2 Real-Time RT-PCR Tests on oral rinses and saliva samples. J Mol Diagn 2021;23:3–9.

26. Hanson KE, Barker AP, Hillyard DR, et al. Self-collected anterior nasal and saliva specimens versus health care worker-collected nasopharyngeal swabs for the molecular detection of SARS-CoV-2. J Clin Microbiol 2020;58(11):e01824-20.

27. Hanson KE, Caliendo AM, Arias CA, et al. The infectious diseases society of America guidelines on the diagnosis of COVID-19: molecular diagnostic testing. Clin Infect Dis 2021. https://doi.org/10.1093/cid/ciab048.

28. Dien Bard J, McElvania E. Panels and syndromic testing in clinical microbiology. Clin Lab Med 2020;40:393–420.

29. Wolters F, van de Bovenkamp J, van den Bosch B, et al. Multi-center evaluation of cepheid xpert(R) xpress SARS-CoV-2 point-of-care test during the SARS-CoV-2 pandemic. J Clin Virol 2020;128:104426.

30. Smith DM, May SJ, Perez-Santiago J, et al. The use of pooled viral load testing to identify antiretroviral treatment failure. AIDS 2009;23:2151–8.

31. Bateman AC, Mueller S, Guenther K, et al. Assessing the dilution effect of specimen pooling on the sensitivity of SARS-CoV-2 PCR tests. J Med Virol 2021;93: 1568–72.

32. Hogan CA, Sahoo MK, Pinsky BA. Sample pooling as a strategy to detect community transmission of SARS-CoV-2. JAMA 2020;323:1967–9.

33. Gwinn M, MacCannell D, Armstrong GL. Next-generation sequencing of infectious pathogens. JAMA 2019;321:893–4.

34. Quainoo S, Coolen JPM, van Hijum S, et al. Whole-genome sequencing of bacterial pathogens: the future of nosocomial outbreak analysis. Clin Microbiol Rev 2017;30:1015–63.

35. Available at: https://www.cdc.gov/amd/how-it-works/detecting-outbreaks-wgs. html. Accessed December 15, 2021.

36. Drake JW, Holland JJ. Mutation rates among RNA viruses. Proc Natl Acad Sci U S A 1999;96:13910–3.

37. Davies NG, Jarvis CI, Group CC-W, et al. Increased mortality in community-tested cases of SARS-CoV-2 lineage B.1.1.7. Nature 2021;593:270–4.

38. Volz E, Mishra S, Chand M, et al. Assessing transmissibility of SARS-CoV-2 lineage B.1.1.7 in England. Nature 2021;593:266–9.

39. Available at: https://www.gov.uk/government/publications/investigation-of-novel-sars-cov-2-variant-variant-of-concern-20201201. Accessed December 15, 2021.

40. Available at: https://www.fda.gov/media/146171/download. Accessed December 15, 2021.

41. Available at: https://www.cdc.gov/coronavirus/2019-ncov/variants/variant-info. html#Interest. Accessed December 15, 2021.

42. Available at: https://www.who.int/en/activities/tracking-SARS-CoV-2-variants/. Accessed December 15, 2021.

43. Buschang PH, LaPalme L, Tanguay R, et al. The technical reliability of superimposition on cranial base and mandibular structures. Eur J Orthod 1986;8:152–6.

44. Chow K, Aslam A, McClure T, et al. Risk of healthcare-associated transmission of SARS-CoV-2 in hospitalized cancer patients. Clin Infect Dis 2021. https://doi.org/ 10.1093/cid/ciab670.

45. Paltansing S, Sikkema RS, de Man SJ, et al. Transmission of SARS-CoV-2 among healthcare workers and patients in a teaching hospital in The Netherlands confirmed by whole-genome sequencing. J Hosp Infect 2021;110:178–83.

46. Planas D, Veyer D, Baidaliuk A, et al. Reduced sensitivity of SARS-CoV-2 variant Delta to antibody neutralization. Nature 2021;596:276–80.
47. Wang H, Jean S, Eltringham R, et al. Mutation-specific SARS-CoV-2 PCR Screen: rapid and accurate detection of variants of concern and the identification of a newly emerging variant with spike L452R mutation. J Clin Microbiol 2021;59: e0092621.
48. Wang H, Miller JA, Verghese M, et al. Multiplex SARS-CoV-2 genotyping reverse transcriptase PCR for population-level variant screening and epidemiologic surveillance. J Clin Microbiol 2021;59:e0085921.
49. Chiara M, D'Erchia AM, Gissi C, et al. Next generation sequencing of SARS-CoV-2 genomes: challenges, applications and opportunities. Brief Bioinform 2021;22: 616–30.
50. Greninger AL, Dien Bard J, Colgrove RC, et al. Clinical and infection prevention applications of SARS-CoV-2 genotyping: an IDSA/ASM consensus review document. Clin Infect Dis 2021. https://doi.org/10.1093/cid/ciab761.
51. Available at: https://www.gisaid.org/. Accessed December 15, 2021.
52. Hadfield J, Megill C, Bell SM, et al. Nextstrain: real-time tracking of pathogen evolution. Bioinformatics 2018;34:4121–3.
53. Available at: https://cov-lineages.org/resources/pangolin.html. Accessed December 15, 2021.
54. Available at: https://nextstrain.org/. Accessed December 15, 2021.
55. Rambaut A, Holmes EC, O'Toole A, et al. A dynamic nomenclature proposal for SARS-CoV-2 lineages to assist genomic epidemiology. Nat Microbiol 2020;5: 1403–7.
56. Available at: https://www.fda.gov/media/135659/download. Accessed December 15, 2021.
57. Gorzalski AJ, Tian H, Laverdure C, et al. High-Throughput Transcription-mediated amplification on the Hologic Panther is a highly sensitive method of detection for SARS-CoV-2. J Clin Virol 2020;129:104501.
58. Available at: https://www.cdc.gov/coronavirus/2019-ncov/lab/resources/antigen-tests-guidelines.html. Accessed December 15, 2021.
59. Prince-Guerra JL, Almendares O, Nolen LD, et al. Evaluation of Abbott Binax-NOW rapid antigen test for SARS-CoV-2 infection at two community-based testing sites - pima county, Arizona, november 3-17, 2020. MMWR Morb Mortal Wkly Rep 2021;70:100–5.
60. Pollock NR, Jacobs JR, Tran K, et al. Performance and implementation evaluation of the abbott BinaxNOW rapid antigen test in a high-throughput drive-through community testing site in Massachusetts. J Clin Microbiol 2021;59:e00083-21.
61. Jaaskelainen AE, Ahava MJ, Jokela P, et al. Evaluation of three rapid lateral flow antigen detection tests for the diagnosis of SARS-CoV-2 infection. J Clin Virol 2021;137:104785.
62. Allan-Blitz LT, Klausner JD. A real-world comparison of SARS-CoV-2 rapid antigen testing versus PCR testing in Florida. J Clin Microbiol 2021;59:e0110721.
63. Hanson KE, Altayar O, Caliendo AM, et al. The infectious diseases society of America guidelines on the diagnosis of COVID-19: antigen testing. Clin Infect Dis 2021. https://doi.org/10.1093/cid/ciab557.
64. Available at: https://www.nytimes.com/2020/04/27/opinion/biomedical-national-guard-covid.html. Accessed December 15, 2021.
65. Wu J, Liu X, Liu J, et al. Coronavirus disease 2019 test results after clinical recovery and hospital discharge among patients in China. JAMA Netw Open 2020;3: e209759.

66. Available at: https://www.cdc.gov/coronavirus/2019-ncov/testing/diagnostic-testing.html. Accessed December 15, 2021.
67. Rhee C, Kanjilal S, Baker M, et al. Duration of severe acute respiratory syndrome coronavirus 2 (SARS-CoV-2) Infectivity: when is it safe to discontinue isolation? Clin Infect Dis 2021;72:1467–74.
68. Storch GA. Diagnostic virology. Clin Infect Dis 2000;31:739–51.
69. Singanayagam A, Patel M, Charlett A, et al. Duration of infectiousness and correlation with RT-PCR cycle threshold values in cases of COVID-19, England, January to May 2020. Euro Surveill 2020;25(32):2001483.
70. Hogan CA, Huang C, Sahoo MK, et al. Strand-specific reverse transcription PCR for detection of replicating SARS-CoV-2. Emerg Infect Dis 2021;27:632–5.
71. Perera R, Tso E, Tsang OTY, et al. SARS-CoV-2 virus culture and subgenomic RNA for respiratory specimens from patients with mild coronavirus disease. Emerg Infect Dis 2020;26:2701–4.
72. Truong TT, Ryutov A, Pandey U, et al. Increased viral variants in children and young adults with impaired humoral immunity and persistent SARS-CoV-2 infection: a consecutive case series. EBioMedicine 2021;67:103355.
73. Alexandersen S, Chamings A, Bhatta TR. SARS-CoV-2 genomic and subgenomic RNAs in diagnostic samples are not an indicator of active replication. Nat Commun 2020;11:6059.
74. Available at: https://www.who.int/publications/i/item/WHO-2019-nCoV-lab-testing-2021.1-eng. Accessed December 15, 2021.

An Overview of SARS-CoV-2 Molecular Diagnostics in Europe

Emma Davies, BSc, MSc, DClinSci, FRCPath[a],*,
Hamzah Z. Farooq, MBChB, MRCP, MSc, DipRCPath[a,b],
Benjamin Brown, BSc, MSc, PhD[a], Peter Tilston, BSc, MSc[a],
Ashley McEwan, BSc, MSc[a], Andrew Birtles, BSc, MSc, PhD[a],
Robert William O'Hara, BSc, PGCert, MSc, PhD, FIBMS[a],
Shazaad Ahmad, BMedSci, BMBS, MSc, FRCPath[a],
Nicholas Machin, BMedSci, BMBS, MSc, FRCPath[a],
Louise Hesketh, BSc, PhD, FRCPath[a], Malcolm Guiver, BSc, PhD, FRCPath[a]

KEYWORDS

- SARS-CoV-2 • COVID-19 • RT-PCR • Molecular diagnostics • CE Marking

KEY POINTS

- The COVID-19 pandemic has led not only to an influx of new molecular diagnostics but also a drive to modify existing technologies to allow the testing of thousands of patients daily over a variety of settings.
- The need for rapid turn-around times for severe acute respiratory syndrome coronavirus-2 (SARS-CoV-2) testing for public health actions and patient care has led to the necessity for synchronously using multiple assays and platforms.
- Testing solutions exist for any scale of SARS-CoV-2 testing strategy.
- Overall SARS-CoV-2 molecular diagnostics seem to perform well; however, market saturation has left peer-reviewed real-world data lacking.
- With these new developments, diagnostic testing regulations for SARS-CoV-2 are paramount to aid manufacturers in achieving assay performance and for laboratories to use as a tool alongside local verification to determine the suitability of assays and platforms for use in future epidemics.

Funding: None declared.
Conflict of interest: None declared.
[a] Department of Virology, UK Health Security Agency, Manchester Foundation Trust, Oxford Road, Manchester M13 9WL, UK; [b] Department of Infectious Diseases and Tropical Medicine, North Manchester General Hospital, Manchester Foundation Trust, Manchester, UK
* Corresponding author. Department of Virology, UK Health Security Agency, Manchester Foundation Trust, Oxford Road, Manchester M13 9WL, UK.
E-mail address: emma.davies@mft.nhs.uk

INTRODUCTION

An emerging viral pneumonia of unknown etiology was detected in patients from several health care facilities in the city of Wuhan in China on 30 December 2019.[1] A novel coronavirus was identified initially termed "2019-nCoV" and designated as severe acute respiratory syndrome coronavirus-2 (SARS-CoV-2) with the clinical disease termed "coronavirus infectious disease-19" (COVID-19).[2–5] It has overwhelmed health care systems globally due to rapid asymptomatic spread and lethality leading the World Health Organization (WHO) to declare a COVID-19 pandemic on 11 March 2020.[6–8]

CLASSIFICATION OF SEVERE ACUTE RESPIRATORY SYNDROME CORONAVIRUS-2, VIRION, AND GENOME

SARS-CoV-2 is a betacoronavirus and one of the seven known members of the Coronaviridae family.[4,9] It is an enveloped positive-strand RNA virus (single linear RNA segment) with a genome length of 29,881 bp (GenBank no. MN908947). Its genome has 14 open reading frames (ORFs), which encode for 28 different proteins—4 structural proteins such as the S (spike), E (envelope), M (membrane), and N (nucleocapsid) proteins; 16 nonstructural proteins (NSP 1–16); and 8 accessory proteins as shown in **Table 1**.[10]

The genome commences with a 5′ untranslated region (UTR), then the replication complex (ORF1a and ORF1b) followed by the four structural proteins and 3′ UTR, ending with nonstructural ORFs and a poly(A) tail.[10,11] ORF1a contains 10 NSPs, while ORF1b contains 16 NSPs. The combination of ORF1a and ORF1b codes for polyproteins pp1a and pp1b that form the viral replication complex.[10,11] Structurally, the RNA genome is bound by the N protein, while the S, E, and M proteins together create the double-layered lipid viral envelope. The principle genes of diagnostic significance are the RdRp (NSP-12), various ORF1ab regions, and the viral structural proteins (S, E, and N).[10]

HISTORY OF SEVERE ACUTE RESPIRATORY SYNDROME CORONAVIRUS-2 MOLECULAR DIAGNOSTICS

The early sequencing of the SARS-CoV-2 genome and subsequent distribution of the genome sequence via Global Initiative on Sharing Avian Influenza Data (GISAID) enabled the development of nucleic acid amplification tests (NAATs), which became the cornerstone for the diagnosis of SARS-CoV-2. Although that is not the only molecular diagnostic technique, real-time polymerase chain reaction (RT-PCR) has become the mainstay across Europe with only limited use of other molecular techniques such as transcription-mediated amplification (TMA) or CRISPR.[12,13] One of the first published RT-PCR assays originated from Europe in January 2020 with primer probe sets targeting the E, N, and RdRp genes.[14] The RdRp assay included a Pan Sarbecco probe that detected SARS-CoV-1, SARS-CoV-2, and Bat-SARS-related-CoV with a second probe specific to SARS-CoV-2 leading to the recommendation of using the E gene assay as the first-line screening tool, followed by confirmatory testing with the RdRp gene assay.[14] A further assay was quickly developed by the Centers for Disease Control and Prevention (CDC) targeting multiple regions of the N gene, which has become the baseline assay for several commercially available molecular diagnostic tests.[15–18]

DIAGNOSTIC TESTING REGULATIONS IN EUROPE

At the start of the COVID pandemic, in vitro medical devices (IVD), including NAAT-based systems and assays, needed to comply with European Union Directive 98/79/EC In Vitro

Table 1
Table showing SARS-CoV-2 structural and nonstructural proteins and their respective functions

Gene	Protein	Function	References
Structural protein			
Spike (S)	S	Binds to Angiotensin-Converting Enzyme 2 (ACE2) receptor and heparan sulfate for viral entry	111
Envelope (E)	E	Virion structure	112
Membrane (M)	M	Virion structure	112
Nucleocapsid (N)	N	Contains genome; interferes with translation and cell cycle of the host cell.	113
Nonstructural protein (NSP)			
ORF1a *ORF1b*	NSP-1	RNA processing and replication	114
	NSP-2	Modulation of survival signaling pathway of host cell	115
	NSP-3	Possibly separates translated protein	116
	NSP-4	Contains transmembrane domain 2 (TM2) and modifies ER membranes	117
	NSP-5	Polyprotein replication	118
	NSP-6	Presumptive transmembrane domain	119
	NSP- 7 and NSP-8	Increases the combination of NSP-12 and template-primer RNA	120
	NSP-9	ssRNA-binding protein	120
	NSP-10	Cap methylation of viral mRNAs	121
	NSP-11	Unknown	122
	NSP-12	RNA-dependent RNA polymerase (RdRp)	123
	NSP-13	Binds with ATP and the zinc-binding domain - required for replication and transcription	124
	NSP-14	Proofreading exoribonuclease domain	125
	NSP-15	Mn(2+)-dependent endoribonuclease activity	126
	NSP-16	2'-O-ribose methyltransferase	127
	ORF 3a	Ion channel protein—affected cytokine response	128
	ORF 6	Inhibits antiviral interferon response	129
	ORF 7a	Inhibits antiviral interferon response and STAT1 phosphorylation	130
	ORF 7b	Inhibits antiviral interferon response, STAT1, and STAT2 phosphorylation	121
	ORF 8	Inhibits antiviral interferon response	131

This table also breaks down the components of *orf1ab* complex.
(*Adapted from* Suryawanshi and colleagues 122 (2021) and Wang and colleagues 132 (2020)).

Diagnostic Directive (IVDD) and bear a **Conformitè Europëenne (**CE) symbol as proof, to be marketed in European Union (EU) and European Free Trade Association countries and Turkey and the United Kingdom.[19,20] CE marking required the manufacturer to have verified compliance with legal requirements and prepared an EC declaration of conformity containing the device performance and safety data.[21] This allowed the device to be CE marked if it was intended for use by health care professionals although specific national requirements may also have been required.[19] Although the United Kingdom left the EU in 2020, it will still accept CE-marked kits until 2023 when the UK Conformity Assessed mark will be required to market IVDs in the United Kingdom.[22] Under Directive 98/79/EC, devices could also be granted emergency market access in the interest of health protection, such as in the COVID-19 pandemic; this required a derogation to be issued by the competent authority of a country allowing temporary marketing of a device without a full declaration of conformity, which was valid only for that nation.[19,21]

As of May 2021, Directive 98/79/EC was replaced in the EU by Regulation (EU) 2017/746, which expands the risk-based device classification system alongside a requirement for device assessment by independent third parties and confirmation of test performance by EU reference laboratories before a CE mark is awarded.[23] All products currently on the market that comply with the old legislation will have to recertify according to the new regulations.[23,24] Regulation (EU) 2017/746 still allows the national emergency market access of IVDs in the interest of protection of health if the derogation is issued by the country's competent authority.[23] This change in regulation brings CE marking more in line with the more stringent Food and Drug Administration (FDA) approval process, which requires devices to be tested by clinical trial and licensed only for use in specific circumstances.[25] On 17 June 2021, the UK government announced the intention to introduce a mandatory validation scheme initially for COVID-19 diagnostics to expand to cover all devices sold in the United Kingdom. This process would require manufacturers to provide a minimum set of standard performance data, which would undergo independent verification by specially commissioned laboratories. If successfully introduced, it would be a criminal offense to market devices that have failed or not undergone this mandatory validation in the United Kingdom under the Medicines and Medical Devices Act 2021.[26]

The above pieces of legislation along with the European Commission's guidelines for the Current Performance of COVID-19 Test Methods and Devices and Proposed Performance Criteria state the performance characteristics for IVDs, which includes but is not limited to analytical and diagnostic sensitivity and specificity, limits of detection (LODs), and expected values in normal and affected populations.[19,23,27] No required values for these characteristics are published in these documents although common specifications are planned.[24] A list of CE-marked COVID-19 IVDs is maintained at the European commission's Joint Research Centre In Vitro Diagnostic Devices and Test Methods Database.[28] As of 08/06/2021 325 CE-marked NAATs exist in this database originating from 240 unique manufacturers with 31 countries of origin. This database lacks key performance criteria for a significant number of entries including 120 tests with no stated LOD, 226 with no analytical sensitivity, 209 with no analytical specificity, and 200 with no clinical accuracy data. The entrance of many nontraditional manufacturers to the market has fueled a lack of peer-reviewed publications that make assessment of real-world performance difficult. An improved and standardized approach to market regulations would be welcomed as at present local validations/verifications of diagnostics are hugely important in ensuring the suitability of test selection for the intended purpose.

In addition to CE marking, the WHO and national bodies such as the UK Medicines and Healthcare products Regulatory Agency (MHRA) have published target product profiles (TPPs) that outline performance characteristics that a test must meet to be considered successful for its intended use.[29–32] WHO and MHRA TPPs outline "acceptable" and "desirable" characteristics including ranges for parameters such as analytical sensitivity/LOD and clinical sensitivity.[29–31] These documents are not legally binding but were developed to aid manufacturers in achieving assay performance that would be desired for use in the field. Equally these documents can be used by laboratories as a tool alongside local verification to determine the suitability of an assay for use. A selection of characteristics for NAAT-based tests is listed in **Tables 2** and **3** with the MHRA TPP showing much stricter acceptable criteria than the WHO criteria recommended for adoption by European Centre for Disease Prevention and Control (ECDC).[29–31,33]

SEVERE ACUTE RESPIRATORY SYNDROME CORONAVIRUS-2 MOLECULAR DIAGNOSTICS

The scale of testing required to manage the SARS-COV-2 pandemic has been unprecedented with extensive yet flexible testing strategies being key to protecting public health through prompt isolation of cases.[33,34] The United Kingdom has undertaken a dual-arm approach to testing with twice weekly at home rapid antigen tests being freely available and actively encouraged in the asymptomatic general population and in laboratory NAAT being used for more sensitive screening of all hospital admissions including day case and those with symptoms consistent with COVID-19.[35,36] The ECDC not only recommends the use of NAAT for all symptomatic cases but also acknowledges the role for rapid antigen tests in population screening.[33,34] The use of sensitive molecular diagnostic assays is important to the control of transmission. If SARS-CoV-2 infection is allowed to spread unchecked, the emergence of novel variants is likely to be enhanced as mutations in key genes continue to accumulate as part of the natural error-prone replication of RNA viruses. As mutations accumulate, it is not only possible that they can lead to increased pathogenicity or vaccine escape, but that they may also lead to detection failures in well-established diagnostic assays. It is now recommended that the presence of SARS-CoV-2 in clinical samples is determined through the detection of at least two distinct targets to mitigate this risk. The observation of the ThermoFisher S gene PCR assay failure in the United Kingdom for the B.1.1.7 Alpha variant, which would have led to significant numbers of false-negative tests being reported if this was being used as a single target assay, highlights the importance of a multi-target approach.[37]

To achieve testing on such an immense scale testing, a diverse approach has been required with laboratories often using multiple assays and platforms in unison. The following is by no means an extensive review of all diagnostic assays used in Europe but aims to provide an overview of some of the most common. Rapid antigen near patient point of care and isothermal amplification techniques are outside the scope of this review but will be covered elsewhere in this Clinics edition.

RAPID MOLECULAR DIAGNOSTICS

Rapid, commercial, cartridge-based sample-to-answer molecular diagnostic platforms for the detection of SARS-CoV-2 have fulfilled an important niche in point-of-care settings and clinical laboratories. They are simple to use, provide accurate results within 1–2 h, have minimal hands-on time, and permit on-demand testing of urgent specimens.

Table 2
Selected target product profile characteristics for point-of-care SAR-CoV-2 detection tests

Scope	World Health Organization		Medicines and Healthcare Products Regulatory Agency	
	Desired	Acceptable	Desired	Acceptable
Intended use	In areas with confirmed SAR-CoV-2 community-wide transmission. In suspected outbreak situations and to monitor trends in disease incidence.		Aid in the triage of current SARS-CoV-2 infection during active infection.	Aid in the triage of current SARS-CoV-2 infection during the acute phase of infection.
Target population	Patients with acute or subacute respiratory symptoms; suspicious symptoms and contact with confirmed or probable case/living in the area of cluster/community transmission.		People with/without SARS-CoV-2 clinical signs and symptoms if testing appropriate.	People with clinical signs and symptoms associated with SAR-CoV-2 infection.
Target user/settings	Trained staff in health care facilities or community level or self-administrated.	Trained staff in health care facilities.	Trained health care professional (governed by professional standards authority). In primary/secondary/community health care settings and nonhealth care settings.	
Target analyte	SARS-CoV-2 only biomarker, for example, RNA, protein/antigen.	SARS-CoV-2 only biomarker. Assumption SARS-CoV-1 not circulating	Dual (or more) SARS-CoV-2 RNA or antigen targets.	Single (or more) SARS-CoV-2 RNA or antigen target.
Target type	Anterior nares, saliva/oral fluid, sputum	NP or OP or nasal swab, nasal wash, sputum	Sputum, saliva, or other method not using invasive swab	NP or OP, lower respiratory tract aspirate, BAL, nasopharyngeal wash/aspirate or nasal aspirate
Clinical sensitivity	≥90%	≥80%	>97% within confidence intervals of 93–100% [a]	>80% within 95% confidence intervals of 93–100%[a]
Clinical specificity	≥99%	≥97%	>99% within confidence intervals of 97–100%[b]	>95% within 95% confidence intervals of 90–100%[b]
Analytical sensitivity (LOD)	1×10^4 copies per ml or Ct≈>30	1×10^6 copies per ml or Ct ≈ 25–30	<100 SARS-CoV-2 copies/ml	<1000 SARS-CoV-2 copies/ml
Technical Failure rate	≤ 0.5%	< 2%	< 1%	< 5%
Turnaround time	≤ 20 min	≤ 40 min	< 30 min	< 2 h
Throughput	≥ 10/h per operator	≥ 5/h per operator	> 100 tests per unit per 12 h	> 6 tests per unit per 12 h

Abbreviations: BAL, bronchoalveolar; LOD, limit of detection; NP, nasopharyngeal swab; OP, oropharyngeal swab; Ct, Cycle threshold.
[a] Determined using at least 150 positive clinical samples covering a clinically meaningful range of viral loads.
[b] Determined using at least 250 negative clinical samples.

Table 3
Selected target product profile characteristics for high- and low-throughput diagnostic SAR-CoV-2 detection testing

Scope	World Health Organization		Medicines and Healthcare Products Regulatory Agency	
	Desired	Acceptable	Desired	Acceptable
Intended use	To detect the presence of virus components to diagnose or confirm acute and subacute SARS-CoV-2 infection.		Multiplex—determining current infection by detecting SARS-CoV-2 virus, differentiate other respiratory infections.	Determining current infection by detecting SARS-CoV-2 virus.
Target population	Patients with acute or subacute respiratory symptoms; suspicious symptoms and contact with confirmed or probable case/living in the area of cluster/community transmission.		People with/without clinical signs associated with SARS-CoV-2 infection.	People with clinical signs associated with SAR-CoV-2 infection.
Target settings/ users	High volume: reference laboratories/district hospitals/mobile laboratories. Laboratory technicians. Low volume: outpatient clinics, point of care or near-patient settings. Laboratory technicians/health care workers.		Health care and medical laboratories. Trained health care professional (governed by professional standards authority) and suitably trained and assessed lab technician or scientist.	
Target analyte	Must have at least one target specific for SARS-CoV-2 RNA or protein/antigen.		Dual (or more) SARS-CoV-2 RNA. Multiplex panel for a range of infectious respiratory viruses.	Single SARS-CoV-2 RNA.
Target type	Samples amenable to self-collection: saliva/oral fluid, stool; inactivated samples.	NP or OP or nasal swab. Washes-nasal, oropharyngeal, BAL. Sputum	Oral fluid	NP or OP, lower respiratory tract aspirate, BAL, nasopharyngeal wash/aspirate, or nasal aspirate.
Clinical sensitivity	$\geq$98%	$\geq$95%	>99%. 95% two-sided confidence interval > 97%[a]	>95%. 95% two-sided confidence interval > 90%[a]
Clinical specificity	$\geq$99%	$\geq$99%	>99%. 95% two-sided confidence interval > 97%[b]	>95%. 95% two-sided confidence interval > 90%[b]
Analytical sensitivity (LOD)	1×10^2 copies per ml in upper/lower respiratory tract specimens, stool	1×10^3 copies per ml in any respiratory tract specimen.	$\leq$100 SARS-CoV-2 copies/ml	$\leq$1000 SARS-CoV-2 copies/ml

(continued on next page)

Table 3
(continued)

Scope	World Health Organization		Medicines and Healthcare Products Regulatory Agency	
	Desired	Acceptable	Desired	Acceptable
Technical failure rate	NA	NA	<0.2%	<1%
Turnaround time	< 45 min	< 4 h	< 90 min	< 5 h
Throughput	High volume: 200–500 tests in 4 h. Low Volume: 6 patients in 45 min	High volume: 50–150 tests in 4 h. Low volume: 1–4 patients per 45 min	> 200 tests in unit per 4 h	> 50 tests in unit per 4 h

Abbreviations: BAL, bronchoalveolar; LOD, limit of detection; NP, nasopharyngeal swab; OP, oropharyngeal swab.
[a] Determined using at least 150 positive clinical samples covering a clinically meaningful range of viral loads.
[b] Determined using at least 250 negative clinical samples.

Table 4
An overview of rapid, cartridge-based, sample to answer SARS-CoV-2 molecular tests

Test Name	Manufacturer	Target 1	Target 2	Internal Control	Platform	Maximum Sample Capacity	Platform Run Time (min)	Sample Input Volume (uL)
Xpert Xpress SARS-CoV-2 Xpert Xpress SARS-CoV-2/Flu/RSV	Cepheid	N2	E	Manufacturer SPC	GeneXpert Dx and GeneXpert Infinity	2–16 (Dx) or Up to 80 (Infinity)	45	300
BioFire® Respiratory Panel 2.1 plus (RP2.1 plus)	BioMerieux	S	M	Schizosaccharomyces pombe	FilmArray 2.0 and FilmArray Torch	2–12	45	300
Cobas Liat SARS-CoV-2 and Influenza A/B	Roche	ORF1 a/b	N	Manufacturer SPC	Cobas Liat	1	20	200
Novodiag COVID-19	MobiDiag	ORF1 a/b	N	RNAse P and Manufacturer SPC	Novodiag	4–16	60	500
VitaPCR SARS-CoV-2 VitaPCR SARS-CoV-2/Flu AB	Credo Diagnostics Biomedical Pte	N	N	β-globin	VitaPCR	1	20	30[a]
Aries SARS-CoV-2	Luminex	ORF1a/b	N	RNAse P	Aries	12	120	200
GenomEra SARS-CoV-2 GenomEra SARS-CoV-2, Flu A/B+ RSV	Abacus Diagnostica	RdRP	E[b]	MS2	GenomEra CDX	4	70	35[c]
QIAstat-Dx Respiratory SARS-CoV-2 Panel	Qiagen	ORF1 a/b (RdRp)	E	MS2	QIAstat Dx Analyzer	1	70	300
GenMark ePlex SARS-CoV-2 GenMark ePlex Respiratory Pathogen Panel 2 (RP2)	GenMark Dx	N	N	Manufacturer SPC	ePlex	3 (ePlex NP) to 24 (ePlex 4 Tower)	90	200

Abbreviations: N, nucleocapsid; E, envelope protein; S, spike glycoprotein; M, membrane protein; ORF1 a/b, open reading frame 1 a/b; RdRP, RNA-dependent RNA polymerase; SPC, sample process control.

[a] 30 uL lysate (lysis buffer containing sample).

[b] GenomEra SARS-CoV-2 contains E gene. GenomEra SARS-CoV-2, Flu A/B+ RSV contains only RdRP.

[c] 50 uL of sample is heated and mixed with 1 mL of lysis buffer, after which 35 uL of processed sample is loaded onto the test chip.

An overview of the main sample-to-answer platforms is presented in **Table 4**. These single-use tests often automate nucleic acid extraction, purification, amplification, detection, and interpretation of results. All the platforms presented are internally controlled yet only three use an endogenous sample control, which monitors for an adequately taken sample and sample degradation. Independent studies evaluating the performance of rapid RT-PCR tests have varied with few head-to-head comparisons although evaluations of these platforms are more extensively published due to their widespread use in non-specialist laboratories.

Unlike other applications, the rapid testing platforms exhibit significant variation in the technologies used. Cepheid Xpert Xpress, QiaStatDx, and VitaPCR SARS-CoV-2 rely on classic multiplex RT-PCR. Novodiag COVID-19[38] is unique in its use of qPCR and microarray technology for the detection of SARS-CoV-2. GenomEra SARS-CoV-2[39] and GenomEra SARS-CoV-2 with Flu A/B+ RSV[40] use multiplex RT-PCR performed on chips. BioFire Respiratory Panel 2.1 plus (RP2.1plus)[41] achieves extensive multiplexing through an initial RT-PCR step before target amplification using numerous monoplex PCR reactions, which are detected using endpoint melt curve analysis. GenMark ePlex SARS-CoV-2[42] and GenMark ePlex Respiratory Pathogen Panel 2 (RP2)[43] use RT-PCR in combination with electrowetting and GenMark's eSensor technology involving electrochemical detection rather than optical detection of fluorescence.

Aside from the variation in technologies, the rapid testing platforms also offer detection of the widest range of pathogens. With the exception of Luminex Aries, SARS-CoV-2 can be detected in isolation or in combination with influenza as a minimum.[44,45] BioFire RP2.1plus[41] detects 23 respiratory pathogens, GenMark ePlex RP2[43] detects 25 respiratory pathogens, and the QIAstat-Dx Respiratory SARS-CoV-2 Panel[46] detects 22 respiratory pathogens.

Xpert Xpress SARS-CoV-2[47] is the most widely evaluated rapid test with a recent systematic review and meta-analysis encompassing 1734 subjects determining a pooled sensitivity of 99% (97–99, 95% CI) and a specificity of 97% (95–98, 95% CI).[48] Reported sensitivities for other platforms range from 90 to 100% with particular issues noted for samples with high cycle threshold (Ct) values in some studies.[45,49–52] Fitoussi and colleagues (2021)[49] found a VitaPCR SARS-CoV-2 sensitivity of 60% for samples that were positive at Ct > 33 using a comparator N gene assay; however, VitaPCR involves no formal RNA extraction and purification that may account for this poor performance.[49] All tests in **Table 4** were shown to be near 100% specific except for the VitaPCR SARS-CoV-2 and QIAstat-Dx.[45,52] The VitaPCR gave a specificity of 94.7% in one study due to its increased sensitivity over the comparator assay, and a second study showed an improved sensitivity of 99%.[45,49] The QIAStat-Dx gave a specificity of 93% compared with a WHO-recommended RT-PCR.[52]

Evaluations often used small sample sets, due to a limited availability of reagents and used various SARS-CoV-2 reference controls, making LOD comparisons difficult. Reported LODs varied from 100 copies/ml for Xpert Xpress SARS-CoV-2 to 3000 genome copy equivalents for the Aries SARS-CoV-2.[53] Several platforms fail to achieve the MHRA TPP "acceptable" LOD criteria of 1000 copies/ml; GenomEra SARS-CoV-2, Flu A/B+ RSV at 2857 copies/mL,[40] Novodiag COVID-19[38] at 1815 copies/mL when using collection devices other than the provided medium nucleic acid amplification test;[54] and both the GenMark ePlex SARS-CoV-2[42] and the QIAstat-Dx Respiratory SARS-CoV-2 Panel[46] at 1000 copies/ml.

The main limitations of the rapid sample-to-answer platforms include their high cost per test and low sample throughput. Moreover, despite their low complexity, rapid platforms are not infallible, and they are sensitive molecular tests that can be compromised without meticulous sample processing and good laboratory practice. Notably, BioFire and ePlex platforms do not output Ct values, meaning there is no indication of SARS-CoV-2 viral burden that can be of interest to the clinician as higher viral loads have been associated with increased SARS-CoV-2 mortality.[55]

STAND-ALONE REAL-TIME POLYMERASE CHAIN REACTION KITS

One of the biggest barriers to the implementation of SARS-CoV-2 testing in non-specialist laboratories early in the pandemic was the availability of the correct equipment to enable the rapid introduction of testing. The solution to this problem for many manufacturers was the rapid introduction to the market of stand-alone assays encompassing kits, which include the reagents necessary for reverse-transcription PCR, including controls, but that are not tied to a specific extraction or PCR platform. They offer flexibility over more "closed" systems as they can potentially be run on existing instrumentation, precluding the requirement for purchasing new and often expensive equipment. Use of such reagents requires more extensive validation than end-to-end systems, and the onus on providing this validation, including sample preparation and the compatibility of any instrumentation with a particular kit, will fall on the individual laboratory. Some suppliers provide details of compatible platforms, but many do not, and it is this lack of data that have allowed many substandard kits to enter the market. Over 200 CE-marked manual RT-PCR kits are listed on the COVID-19 In Vitro Diagnostic Medical Devices database,[28] a selection of which are shown in **Table 5** along with some of their main attributes.[18,56–73]

Kit formats are broadly similar and include minimal necessary reagents (primer/probe mixes, controls). Reagents may be provided either lyophilized or "wet" most commonly in tubes but also as eight-well strips. Although earlier kits relied on a single viral gene target, these have now been largely superseded by dual or triple target assays that focus on some combination of the E, N, S, and Orf1a genes. Although this has made the assays more robust in dealing with the emergence of novel SARS-CoV-2 variants, it has also complicated the interpretation of results when some gene targets fail to amplify. Furthermore, most kits supply an internal control (IC), which may be either endogenous (eg RNase P)[18,58,64,65,71] or exogenous (eg MS2),[62,63,68] which can be used either as full process controls or solely as PCR controls. Some kits include both endogenous and exogenous ICs[72] although some fail to disclose the IC origin.[52,56,57,59,60,67–70,73]

The number of tests per kit ranges from 48 to 4800 allowing for a wide range of throughputs although this will also depend on the number of wells required per sample and whether they are being tested in 96- or 384-well format. Many assays exploiting RT-PCR can typically use up to four different fluorescent reporter dyes, including the IC, but others are not so comprehensively multiplexed and require two or even three wells for each sample. At least one kit (Menarini)[74] uses melt curve analysis in preference to hydrolysis probes, negating the requirement for multiple fluorescent reporter dyes. Although not shown in **Table 5**, many SARS-CoV-2 kits are also formulated as multiplexes with other respiratory viruses, most commonly influenza and respiratory syncytial virus (RSV), for example, Altona,[75] Viasure,[76] and ThermoFisher.[77] This will usually require the addition of an extra well for each sample and/or the use of a single dye for multiple gene targets of the same virus. The actual throughput for these assays will depend heavily on the extraction and PCR equipment chosen for use and the level of automation. Use of an automated end-to-end system like the Roche FLOW could produce in excess of 1000 results in a 24hr period from experience in our local laboratory.

Table 5
An overview of stand-alone RT-PCR suppliers and kits available in the EU. Details are taken from company websites and/or accompanying literature

Supplier	Kit Name	Target 1	Target 2	Target 3	Internal Control	No' of Tests/Kit	Compatible Platforms	Analytical Sensitivity	References
Altona	RealStar® SARS-CoV-2 Virus RT-PCR Kit 1.0	E	S		Manufacturer SPC	384/4800	Bio-Rad CFX96, Bio-Rad CFX96 deep-well, ABI QuantStudio, ABI 7500, Roche LightCyler 480, Qiagen Rotor-Gene Q	E = 0.025 pfu/mL S = 0.014 pfu/mL	56 66 67 68 69 70
Anatolia Geneworks /Launch	Bosphore Novel Coronavirus (2019-nCoV) Detection Kit v4	Orf1ab	N	E	RNAse P	50/100	Not stated	orf1ab = 0.86 copies/ul N = 0.82 copies/ul E = 1.02 copies/ul	71
Biomaxima	SARS-CoV-2 Real-Time PCR LAB-KITTM	Orf1ab	N		Manufacturer SPC	96 (12 × 8 well strips)	"Open PCR systems"	10 copies/reaction	No literature found[a]
BioMerieux	Argene SARS Cov-2 R-Gene	N	RdRp	E	Endogenous (HPRT1) and Manufacturer SPC	120	ABI 7500, ABI QuantStudio5, Roche LightCycler 480, Bio-Rad CFX96, Qiagen Rotor-Gene Q	0.43 TCID50/mL (equivalent to 380 copies/mL).	72
Bio-Rad	Reliance SARS-CoV-2 RT-PCR Assay Kit	N1	N2		RNAse P	200	Bio-Rad CFX96, ABI 7500	125–250 copies/ml	No literature found[a]
Clonit	Quanty COVID-19 v2 (quantitative)	N1	N2		RNAse P	96	ABI 7500, Qiagen Rotor Gene Q, Bio-Rad CFX96	Not stated	No literature found[a]
Clonit	COVID 19 HT Screen (qualitative)	N1	N2		Manufacturer SPC	96	ABI 7500, Qiagen Rotor Gene Q, Bio-Rad CFX96	Not stated	No literature found[a]

Company	Assay	Gene			Internal control	Throughput	Instruments	LOD	References
Euroimmun	EuroRealTime SARS-CoV-2	Orf1ab	N		Manufacturer SPC	25–1000	Roche LightCycler 480, ABI 7500, Bio-Rad CFX 96, Qiagen Rotor-Gene Q, qTower 3	1 copy/ul	73
Genetic Signatures	EasyScreen SARS-CoV-2 Detection Kit	N	E		Manufacturer SPC	96	ABI Quantstudio 5	Not stated	57
IDT	2019-nCov CDC Assay	N1	N2		RNAse P	96	ABI 7500	1–3 copies/ul	18 58
Menarini	Corona MELT	Orf1ab	Orf1ab		Human GADPH	100	Most commercial Real Time PCR instruments	20 copies/reaction	No literature found[a]
Perkin Elmer	SARS-CoV-2 Real-time RT-PCR Assay	Orf1ab	N		MS2	48	Bio-Rad CFX96/385, ABI 7500, ABI QuantStudio, qTower 3	20 copies/ml	No literature found[a]
Primerdesign	genesig® COVID-19 2G Real-Time PCR assay	Orf1ab	S		Manufacturer SPC	96	ABI 7500, Bio-Rad CFX Connect, Roche LightCycler 480, genesig® q32	0.4 copies/ul	69 59 60
RIDA®GENE	SARS-CoV-2	E		E	Manufacturer SPC	100/200	RIDA CYCLER, Roche LightCycler 480, Mx3005P, ABI 7500, Bio-Rad CFX96, Qiagen Rotor-Gene Q	50 copies/reaction	61
Seegene	Allplex 2019-nCOV	RdRp	N	E	Manufacturer SPC	50/100	Roche LightCycler 480 (minimum)	1–4 copies/ul	67 69 70 62
Serosep	Respibio SARS-CoV-2	Not stated			Not stated	96	Roche LightCycler 480, ABI 7500	Not stated	No literature found[a]

(continued on next page)

Table 5
(continued)

Supplier	Kit Name	Target 1	Target 2	Target 3	Internal Control	No' of Tests/Kit	Compatible Platforms	Analytical Sensitivity	References
Thermofisher	TaqPath COVID-19 CE-IVD RT-PCR Kit,	S	N	orf1ab	MS2	Up to 1000 (96- and 384-well format)	ABI 7500, ABI Quantstudio 5	10 genome copy equivalents/ reaction	68 62 63
TIBMOL BIOL	Dual Target SARS	N	E		UBC Human mRNA	96	Roche LightCycler 480	Not stated	64 65
ViaSure (CerTest Biotech)	SARS-CoV-2 Real Time PCR	Orf1ab	N		Not stated	96	"Most open PCR systems"	1–10 copies/ reaction	18
VirCell	SARS-CoV-2 Real Time PCR Kit	N	E		RNAse P	48	"Most open PCR systems"	3–5 copies/ reaction	No literature found[a]

Abbreviations: N, nucleocapsid; E, envelope protein; S, spike glycoprotein; ORF1 a/b, open reading frame 1 a/b; RdRP, RNA-dependent RNA polymerase; SPC, sample process control.

[a] Indicates that using the kit name in combination with either "COVID-19" or "SARS CoV-2" as the search term in PubMed and Google Scholar yielded no significant results.

Owing to the pressure to manufacture diagnostic kits rapidly as the pandemic took hold, much of the technical and clinical validation data used minimal data sets. Unlike the rapid platforms that are in widespread use, peer-reviewed literature is sparse for many stand-alone kits and in some cases completely absent. For those referenced assays in **Table 5**, the LOD was most commonly in the range of 1–20 copies/reaction although this was liable to small variations depending on the extraction and eluate volume and the volume of eluate used in the PCR. When comparisons between kits using clinical samples or External Quality Assurance (EQA) samples were performed, most kits performed comparably with only small variations in results between the Altona,[52,56,66–70] Integrated DNA Technologies (IDT),[18,58] Seegene,[62,67,69,70] Taq-Path,[62,63,68] Viasure,[18] and Tib MolBiol kits.[64,65] Specificity was 100% in virtually all cases.

Stand-alone kits offer a convenient alternative to more closed systems allowing rapid implementation on existing equipment. However, despite a broad agreement in the performance of these assays on clinical specimens, the sheer number of kits available means that in-house validation is essential before implementation as a clinical service.

LOW-THROUGHPUT TESTING PLATFORMS

The use of stand-alone PCR kits is not always an attractive option for laboratories, particularly if the existing molecular diagnostic infrastructure is not in place. Manufacturers identified a niche in the market for automated low-to-medium input end-to-end solutions, which could be easily introduced to laboratories with minimal molecular diagnostic experience. All platforms assessed here use multiplex RT-PCR with all assays containing an IC except the Virokey SARS-CoV-2, which contains neither an endogenous nor manufacturer-provided IC (**Table 6**).[78] False-negative results will not be identified by the failure to include an IC to demonstrate either sample adequacy or PCR failure. The Qiagen NeuMoDx has the best throughput of these systems at 435 samples in 24hr and also has the advantage of being a true random access platform with a quick time to result of only 1hr 25 min.[79]

Peer-reviewed literature for these platforms is significantly lacking over all other investigated areas with most performance data presented here being sourced from the manufacturer's literature. The BD MAX system can use a variety of kits from different manufacturers including SARS-CoV-2 in isolation or with other respiratory pathogens such as influenza. The BD MAX SARS-CoV-2 assays, including the ViaSure SARS-CoV-2 N1 + N2 assay, have repeatedly shown 100% sensitivity but the specificity of greater than 95% both in manufacturers post-market surveillance and in real-world data. Fears around the production of false-positive results led the FDA to release a product notice recommending confirmation of all positive results generated by the BD MAX; however, both of the assessed assays are based on the CDC N gene assay, which has been shown to be highly sensitive.[16,17,80] The Amplidiag COVID-19 assay was highly sensitive showing greater than 98% agreement compared directly with Cobas 6800 SARS-CoV-2. All other assessed platforms as shown in **Table 6** were also found to have acceptable sensitivity and specificity of greater than 96% based on manufacturer's data only.[78,79,81–84]

All assessed platforms were shown to have good analytical sensitivity as outlined in **Table 6** with the exception of Aus Diagnostics SARS-CoV-2, influenza, and RSV, which has an LOD on 2150 to 4325 copies/ml.[82] Real-world testing of the Amplidiag COVID-19 also highlighted a failure to detect an EQA sample at 3300 copies/ml suggesting the manufacturer published LOD of 313 copies/ml may not be reliable.[83] Local

Table 6
An overview of low- to mid-throughput end-to-end testing platforms for SARS-CoV-2

Supplier/ Platform	Assay	Target 1	Target 2	Internal Control	Analytical Sensitivity	Batch Size	Platform Run Time	Throughput 24hr	References
Mobidiag Amplidiag Easy	Amplidiag COVID-19	Orf1	N	RNAse P	313 copies/ml	48	3.5 h	288	133 134 135
BD MAX	BD SARS-CoV-2	N1	N2	RNAse P	640 genomic copy equivalents	24	2.5 h	216	17
EliTech Elite InGenius	SARS-CoV-2 PLUS ELITe MGB Kit	Orf1ab	Orf8	RNAse P	111 genomic copy equivalents	12	2.5 h	108	81
ViaSure (CerTest Biotech)	SARS-CoV-2 (N1 + N2) – BD MAX	N1	N2	RNAse P	$\geq$ 5 genome copies per reaction	24	2.5 h	216	16
Vela Diagnostics Sentosa	ViroKey SARS-CoV-2 RT-PCR Test v2.0	Orf1a	N	None	200 genome equivalents/ml	46	4 h	276	78
Aus Diagnostics HighPlex 24	SARS-CoV-2 influenza and RSV 8-well	Orf1	Orf8	Endogenous and Manufacturer SPC	2150–4325 copies/ml	24	4.5 h	120	82 136
NeuMoDx™	NeuMoDx™ SARS-CoV-2 Assay	Nsp2	N	Manufacturer SPC	200[11]	Random Access	1 h 25 min	435	84

Abbreviations: N, nucleocapsid; ORF1 a/b, open reading frame 1 a/b; Orf 8, open reading frame 8; SPC, sample process control.

verification of the manufacturer's claims is important before the introduction of any test into routine use to ensure discrepancies such as this are detected.

The expected 24hr throughput for these systems is modest, and these systems are likely to be sited in laboratories that do not undertake 24/7 working meaning their full potential cannot be met. Although this may be the case, these automated solutions can offer easy-to-use solutions for laboratories with limited molecular experience. This has been important in providing the ability to decrease time to result over sending samples to specialist reference laboratories for testing, which in turn can reduce transmission risk particularly in health care settings.

HIGH-THROUGHPUT TESTING PLATFORMS

Several high-throughput platforms have been introduced for the detection of SARS-CoV-2 RNA offering end-to-end automated testing of samples from nucleic acid extraction through to amplification and detection. The introduction of high-throughput screening platforms into laboratories can improve laboratory efficiency and turnaround times while reducing staff hands-on time[85] and facilitating a substantial increase in a testing capacity. The main high-throughput testing platforms and associated assays are listed in **Table 7**. All are RT-PCR-based assays except the Hologic Aptima SARS-CoV-2 assay that use TMA. All assays listed use a minimum of two different SARS-CoV-2 targets to reduce the risk of false negatives due to primer/probe mismatches caused by sequence variability.[86] Multiple comparisons between the high-throughput platforms and standard RT-PCR demonstrate a high level of diagnostic performance. The Panther Fusion had an overall agreement of 96.4% compared with the Roche Cobas 6800 SARS-CoV-2 assay[87] with a similar finding in a separate study.[88] An agreement of 98.3% was found when comparing the Cobas to the Abbott Alinity M SARS-CoV-2 AMP,[89] and in a three-way comparison between these platforms and the Panther Fusion, the overall agreement was 99.7%.[90] When the TMA-based Aptima assay was compared with the Panther Fusion and rapid low-throughput BioFire Defense COVID-19 test, it produced a positive percent agreement of 98.7% compared with the consensus and a 100% agreement for negative results.[91]

Comparing analytical sensitivity is difficult due to differences in methods between studies, but generally all have high analytical sensitivities with LODs of 200 copies/ml or below, as collated from several studies and listed in **Table 1**. The TMA-based Aptima assay was shown to have a lower LOD when compared with standard RT-PCR,[13] although when compared directly against the Roche Cobas and Abbott m2000, the Cobas test had the lowest LOD,[84] a similar finding when the Cobas was directly compared with the Abbott m2000 and Panther Fusion.[92]

All systems offer a throughput of 1000 samples or more in a 24hr period. The highest throughput systems are the Roche Cobas 8800 system and the recently introduced Thermofisher Amplitude running the Taqpath COVID-19 assay, which claims a very high throughput of 8000 samples from a single platform over 24 hours. The Taqpath COVID-19 assay has been evaluated as a standard RT-PCR[62] assay, but no published data exist for the diagnostic performance of the complete Amplitude system. Assays for these high-throughput platforms are being updated to include additional respiratory targets to meet the predicted increases in RSV and seasonal influenza infections once nonpharmaceutical interventions for COVID are removed.[93] These include the Roche Cobas SARS-CoV-2 and Influenza A/B for the 6800/800 systems, the Aptima SARS-CoV-2/Flu Assay for the Hologic Panther system, and the m RESP-4-PLEX ASSAY for the Abbott Alinity system.[94] The Cepheid GeneXpert infinity platform can

Table 7
An overview of high-throughput molecular diagnostic platforms for SARS-CoV-2

Platform	Assay	Target 1	Target 2	Target 3	Internal Control	Analytical Sensitivity SARS-CoV-2 RNA c/ml	Platform Run Time	Throughput 24hr	Loading	References
Abbott m2000	Abbott RealTime SARS-CoV-2	RdRp	N		Manufacturer SPC	53[92]	4 h	470	Batch	92
Abbott Alinity M	SARS-CoV-2 AMP Kit	RdRp	N		Manufacturer SPC (DNA)	50[90]	2 h 35 min to first results	1080	Random Access	90
Hologic Panther®	Aptima® SARS-CoV-2 Assay	Orf1Ab Region 1	Orf1ab Region 2		Manufacturer SPC	83–194[137,138]	3.5 h to the first result	1150	Batch	137 138
Hologic Panther Fusion®	Panther Fusion® SARS-CoV-2 Assay	Orf1Ab Region 1	Orf1ab Region 2		Manufacturer SPC	74–100[92,139,140]	2.4 h to first results	1440	Random Access	92 139 140
Roche Cobas® 6800	cobas® SARS-CoV-2	Orf1ab	E		Manufacturer SPC	<10–85[92,141]	3.4 h to first results	1440	Batch	92 141
Roche Cobas® 8800								4128	Batch	
Cepheid Infinity	Xpert Xpress SARS-CoV-2	N	E		Manufacturer SPC	100	50 min per cartridge	Up to 1920	Random Access	95
Thermofisher Amplitude	TaqPath COVID-19 HT	S gene	N	Orf1ab	MS2	N/A	3 h 30 min to first result	8000	Batch	No literature found

give users the option to run up to 80 Xpert Xpress SARS-CoV-2 cartridges simultaneously with no increase in run time over the smaller cepheid instruments making this a high-throughput low complexity solution for laboratory settings.[95]

SEVERE ACUTE RESPIRATORY SYNDROME CORONAVIRUS-2 GENOTYPING

All viruses mutate, particularly RNA viruses, and the infection rate of SARS-Cov-2 on a large susceptible population has greatly increased the opportunity for mutations to occur. These mutations have led to variants of concern (VOCs) emerging with the potential of enhanced fitness, specifically toward increased transmissibility[96,97] and vaccine evasion.[98–102]

The first VOC (B.1.1.7—Alpha) was detected in the south of England and sequenced in September 2020.[103] Soon after, new VOCs were identified from various locations across the world, each VOC becoming a prominent strain within their area of origin.[104] Genomic sequencing is an invaluable tool in managing the pandemic due to its ability to detect unknown variations, which may indicate the emergence of a new VOC and the need for the development of new diagnostic assays. The United Kingdom currently sequences all SARS-CoV-2-positive samples where it is technically achievable; however, it can be slow, technically demanding, and currently has limited global availability.[34] One solution to identifying known SARS-CoV-2 lineages without the need for genomic sequencing is the development of real-time genotyping PCR assays.

Rapid real-time genotyping PCR assays usually target a single nucleotide polymorphism (SNP), with the most discriminatory targets often located within the S-gene. These types of mutations invariably lead to nonsynonymous amino acid substitutions. SNPs within this region can cause changes in the receptor-binding motif with successful variants retaining an increased affinity of the S-protein to the human angiotensin 2 receptor (ACE2).[103,105–107] Identification of these distinct mutations can be used as markers to detect specific VOC lineages.

It is often the case that one distinct mutation may be present in several VOCs. For example, the presence of the N501Y mutation alone can be distinctive of the B.1.1.7 lineage, but the N501Y is also present in the B.1.351 and P1 VOC alongside the E484 K and K417 N or K417 T mutations, respectively; although the E484 K mutation is also occasionally seen in the B.1.1.7 lineage. It is often necessary to assay multiple targets to reliably determine the likely SARS-CoV-2 lineage. The range of SNP assays used will need to be modified as the new VOC are identified through whole-genome sequencing strategies.

Public Health England currently uses the Applied Biosystems (Waltham, Massachusetts, USA) RT-PCR genotyping assay for the rapid detection of variants. This genotyping assay has a sufficient repertoire of target mutations to reliably cover all the major VOC currently recognized by the WHO and most of the variants of interest.[108,109] The current selection consists of 32 assays that can detect 30 SNPs and 2 deletions. Each assay is duplex in format detecting the mutant and the original SARS-CoV-2 reference/wild-type sequence on two different fluorescent dye layers. The high specificity of each assay target results in a significant reduction in the sensitivity, and it is advised by the manufacturer to only use extracted RNA from specimens with a CT of $\leq$30 where this information is available.[109] There are several VOC assays in development or in early stages of marketing as shown in **Table 8**, many of which exist in stand-alone format to allow a reactive and rapid introduction of new SNP assays to the market as dictated by circulating variants. Agena Bioscience has developed the MassARRAY SARS-CoV-2 Variant Panel capable of

Table 8
A small selection of SNP PCR assays available in Europe for the detection of SARS-CoV-2 variants of concern

Manufacturer	Assay	Targets	Variant	References
EliTech	SARS-CoV-2 Variants ELITe MGB® Kit	• S gene, E484 K • S gene, N501Y	Alpha	142
ViaSure (CerTest Biotech)	SARS-CoV-2 & UK Variant	• HV 69/70 s gene deletion	Alpha	143
Anatolia Geneworks/ Launch	Bosphore SARS-CoV-2 UK. Variant Detection Kit	• A570D • P681H • Y144del	Alpha	144

Thermofisher	TaqMan Custom SNP Assays	Bottom of Form
		• D215 G
		• D614 G
		• HV 69/70 s gene deletion
		• Y144del
		• E484 K
		• E484Q
		• F888 L
		• K417 N
		• K417 T
		• L18 F
		• L452 R
		• N439 K
		• N501Y
		• P681H
		• P681 R
		• S13I
		• S477 N
		• T20 N
		• V1176 F
			Alpha
			Beta
			Gamma
			Delta
			Plus numerous
			  variants of
			  interest
			  depending
			  on combination
			  used
				109
				108

TIBMOL BIOL	VirSNiP Assays	• H66D
		• A67 V
		• HV 69/70 s gene deletion
		• D253 G
		• K417 N
		• K417 T
		• L452 R
		• Y453 F
		• T478 K
		• E484 K
		• E484Q
		• N501Y
		• A570D
		• P681H
		• P681 R
		• F888 L
		• Q949 R
		• V1176 F
			Alpha
			Beta
			Gamma
			Delta
			Plus numerous
			  variants of
			  interest
			  depending
			  on combination
			  used
				145

(continued on next page)

Table 8 (continued)				
Manufacturer	**Assay**	**Targets**	**Variant**	**References**
Agena Bioscience	MassARRAY SARS-CoV-2 Variant Panel	• L452 R • E484Q • P681 R • T478 K • T19 R • P681H • N501Y • A570D • HV 69/70 s gene deletion • S982 A • T716I • Y144del • D80 A • D215 G • K417 N • E484 K • A701 V • L18 F • L242_L244del • Q677H • D253 G • L5F • T95I • S477 N • D80 G • S13I • W152 C • N439 K • K1191 N • Q493 K • I692 V • Y453 F • N501 T • Q677P	15 variants of interest including: Alpha Beta Gamma Delta	110

detecting 15 variants over 36 gene targets in a two-well multiplex end-point RT-PCR assay.[110]

The use of SNP genotyping assays for the detection of SARS-CoV-2 VOC can be an effective early warning system for emerging VOC within a population, with quicker turnaround times compared with genomic sequencing. Data produced from this method can help scientists to quickly predict the prevalence of a VOC within a given population and may provide evidence toward vaccine effectiveness for new variants when collated with data regarding new infections or hospitalizations.

SUMMARY

The COVID-19 pandemic will have a long-reaching impact on molecular diagnostic testing. The speed at which molecular diagnostics entered the market has been un-rivaled with strategies suitable for all desired testing throughputs available within a few short months. The overall analytical and clinical accuracy data for solutions marketed within Europe have generally been found to be satisfactory although published LODs can be variable. At the outset of the pandemic manufacturers, claims were not required to be independently verified in Europe, and outside the most used rapid or high-throughput testing platforms, peer-reviewed real-world data are sparse. Welcome changes to regulations for devices in Europe are on the horizon, but local laboratory validations will still play a key role in the future. With the increasing prevalence of new SARS-CoV-2 VOC and the need for enhanced surveillance, there is still potential for new developments in SARS-CoV-2 molecular diagnostics.

CLINICS CARE POINTS

- evere acute respiratory syndrome coronavirus-2 (SARS-CoV-2) required the rapid expansion of virological diagnostic techniques to ensure adequate testing capacity in the pandemic settings.
- Rapid, molecular diagnostic platforms fulfill an important niche in point-of-care settings and clinical laboratories. They provide quick accurate results require minimal hands-on time and permit on-demand testing of urgent specimens, which is pertinent for non-COVID patient care.
- High-throughput platforms improve laboratory efficiency and turnaround times while reducing staff hands-on time. This leads to an increase in the testing capacity of diagnostic laboratories to help meet the clinical demand throughout pandemics.
- The use of SNP genotyping assays for the detection of SARS-CoV-2 VOCs can be an effective early warning system for emerging VOCs within a population, with faster turnaround times compared with genomic sequencing. This can assist with public health surveillance and provide high-quality evidence toward vaccine effectiveness.

REFERENCES

1. ProMED-mail. Published Date : 2020-01-05 18 : 15 : 37 Subject : PRO/AH/EDR > Undiagnosed Pneumonia - China (HU) (03): Updates , SARS , MERS Ruled out , WHO , RFI Archive Number : 20200105 . 6872267.; 2020.
2. Zhang Y-Z. Initial genome release of novel coronavirus. Virological. Available at: https://virological.org/t/novel-2019-coronavirus-genome/319. 2020. Accessed June 23, 2021.
3. World Health Organization. Novel coronavirus (2019-NCoV) situation reports. Available at: https://www.who.int/docs/default-source/coronaviruse/situation-reports/20200121-sitrep-1-2019-ncov.pdf?sfvrsn=20a99c10_4. 2020. Accessed June 23, 2021.
4. Coronaviridae Study Group of the International Committee on Taxonomy of Viruses. The species Severe acute respiratory syndrome-related coronavirus: classifying 2019-nCoV and naming it SARS-CoV-2. Nat Microbiol 2020;5(4): 536–44.
5. World Health Organization. Naming the coronavirus disease (COVID-19) and the virus that causes it. Available at: https://www.who.int/emergencies/diseases/novel-coronavirus-2019/technical-guidance/naming-the-coronavirus-disease-(covid-2019)-and-the-virus-that-causes-it. 2020. Accessed June 23, 2021.
6. Tangcharoensathien V, Bassett MT, Meng Q, et al. Are overwhelmed health systems an inevitable consequence of covid-19? Experiences from China, Thailand, and New York State. BMJ 2021;372:n83.

7. Narain JP, Dawa N, Bhatia R. Health system response to COVID-19 and future pandemics. J Health Manag 2020;22(2):138–45.

8. Cucinotta D, Vanelli M. WHO declares COVID-19 a pandemic. Acta Biomed 2020;91(1):157–60.

9. Huang Y, Yang C, Xu X, et al. Structural and functional properties of SARS-CoV-2 spike protein: potential antivirus drug development for COVID-19. Acta Pharmacol Sin 2020;41(9):1141–9.

10. Wu A, Peng Y, Huang B, et al. Genome composition and divergence of the novel Coronavirus (2019-nCoV) originating in China. Cell Host Microbe 2020;27(3):325–8.

11. Kim D, Lee J-Y, Yang J-S, et al. The architecture of SARS-CoV-2 transcriptome. Cell 2020;181(4):914–21.e10.

12. Datta M, Singh DD, Naqvi AR. Molecular diagnostic tools for the detection of SARS-CoV-2. Int Rev Immunol 2021;40(1–2):143–56.

13. Gorzalski AJ, Tian H, Laverdure C, et al. High-Throughput Transcription-mediated amplification on the Hologic Panther is a highly sensitive method of detection for SARS-CoV-2. J Clin Virol 2020;129(June 2020):104501.

14. Corman VM, Landt O, Kaiser M, et al. Detection of 2019 novel coronavirus (2019-nCoV) by real-time RT-PCR. Euro Surveill 2020;25(3):2000045.

15. Centers for Disease Control and Prevention, CDC 2019-Novel Coronavirus (2019-nCoV) Real-Time RT-PCR Diagnostic Panel. Available at: https://www.fda.gov/media/134922/download. 2020. Accessed June 23, 2021

16. CerTest BioTec. SARS-CoV-2 (N1 + N2) for BD MAXTM System Instructions for Use. Available at: https://www.certest.es/products/sars-cov-2-n1-n2-bd-maxtm-system/. 2021. Accessed June 23, 2021.

17. Becton Dickinson & Company. SARS-CoV-2 Reagents for BD MAX System Instructions for Use. Available at: https://www.fda.gov/media/136816/download. 2020. Accessed June 23, 2021.

18. Freire-Paspuel B, Vega-Mariño P, Velez A, et al. Analytical and clinical comparison of Viasure (CerTest Biotec) and 2019-nCoV CDC (IDT) RT-qPCR kits for SARS-CoV2 diagnosis. Virology 2021;553:154–6.

19. European Commission. Directive 98/79/EC of the European Parliament and of the Council of 27 October 1998 on in Vitro Diagnostic Medical Devices. Vol 75. Available at: https://www.legislation.gov.uk/eudr/1998/79/pdfs/eudr_19980079_1998-12-07_en.pdf. 2003. Accessed June 23, 2021.

20. Stralin M. In which countries is CE marking required? Clever Compliance. Available at: https://support.ce-check.eu/hc/en-us/articles/360014076911-In-which-countries-is-CE-marking-required. 2020. Accessed June 2, 2021

21. European Commission. Q&A on in vitro diagnostic medical device conformity assessment and performance in the context of COVID-19. Available at: https://ec.europa.eu/health/system/files/2021-06/covid-19_ivd-qa_en_0.pdf. 2021. Accessed June 23, 2021

22. Medicines and healthcare products regulatory agency. Regulating medical devices in the UK. 2020. Available at: https://www.gov.uk/guidance/regulating-medical-devices-in-the-uk. Accessed June 28, 2021.

23. European Commission. Regulation (EU) 2017/746 of the European parliament and of the council on in vitro diagnostic medical devices. Off J Eur Union 2017;5(5):117–76.

24. MedTech Europe. Is the IVD Regulation Framework Ready for Class D Devices? Available at: https://www.medtecheurope.org/wp-content/uploads/2020/10/

medtech-europe-reflection-paper-class-d-infrastructure-under-ivdr-transition-october-2020-1.pdf. 2020. Accessed June 23, 2021

25. Mishra S. FDA, CE mark or something else?—thinking fast and slow. Indian Heart J 2017;69(1):1–5.

26. Department of Health and Social care. Private COVID-19 testing validation. 2021. Available at: https://www.gov.uk/government/consultations/private-coronavirus-covid-19-testing-validation/private-covid-19-testing-validation. Accessed June 28, 2021.

27. European Commission. Current performance of COVID-19 test methods and devices and proposed performance criteria. Available at: https://ec.europa.eu/docsroom/documents/40805. 2020. Accessed June 23, 2021

28. European Commission. European commission COVID-19 in vitro diagnostic devices and test methods database. 2020. Available at: https://covid-19-diagnostics.jrc.ec.europa.eu. Accessed June 28.

29. World Health Organization. COVID-19 target product profiles for priority diagnostics to support response to the COVID-19 pandemic v.1.0. World Health Organization; 2020.

30. Medicines and Healthcare products Regulatory Agency. Target product profile: point of care SARS-CoV-2 detection tests 2020. https://doi.org/10.1093/med/9780199609147.003.0077.

31. Medicines and Healthcare products Regulatory Agency. Target product profile: laboratory-based SARS-CoV-2 viral detection tests 2020. https://doi.org/10.1093/med/9780199609147.003.0077.

32. Medicines and Healthcare products Regulatory Agency. Guidance For industry and manufacturers: COVID-19 tests and testing kits. Available at: https://www.gov.uk/government/publications/how-tests-and-testing-kits-for-coronavirus-covid-19-work/for-industry-and-manufactures-covid-19-tests-and-testing-kits. 2021. Accessed June 23, 2021

33. European Centre for Disease Prevention and Control. COVID-19 testing strategies and objectives key messages. Available at: https://www.ecdc.europa.eu/sites/default/files/documents/TestingStrategy_Objective-Sept-2020.pdf. 2020. Accessed June 23, 2021

34. Royal College of Pathologists, COVID-19 testing, 2020, A National Strategy. Available at: https://www.rcpath.org/profession/on-the-agenda/covid-19-testing-a-national-strategy.html. 2020. Accessed June 23, 2021.

35. Torjesen I. Covid-19: how the UK is using lateral flow tests in the pandemic. BMJ 2021;372:1–3.

36. UK Parliament. Mass asymptomatic Covid-19 testing: strategy and accuracy. 2021. Available at: https://commonslibrary.parliament.uk/research-briefings/cbp-9223/. Accessed June 28, 2021.

37. Public Health England. Investigation of novel SARS-COV-2 variant Variant of Concern 202012/01 Detection of an epidemiological cluster associated with a new variant of concern Nomenclature of variants in the UK Current epidemiological findings. 2020;(December):1-11.

38. MobiDiag. Complete solution for rapid molecular diagnostics of coronavirus infection. Available at: https://mobidiag.com/products/coronavirus/#Novodiag-COVID-19. 2021. Accessed June 14, 2021.

39. Abacus Diagnostica. GenomEra SARS-CoV-2 Assay Kit Package Insert. Available at: https://www.abacusdiagnostica.com/products/sars-cov-2-2-0/. 2020. Accessed June 23, 2021.

40. Abacus Diagnostica. GenomEra SARS-CoV-2 , Flu A/B + RSV Assay Kit Package Insert. Version 1.0. Available at: https://www.abacusdiagnostica.com/products/sars-cov-2-flu-a-b-rsv/. 2020. Accessed June 23, 2021

41. BioFire respiratory Panel 2.1 plus (RP2.1plus) Instructions for use. Available at: https://www.biomerieux-diagnostics.com/filmarrayr-respiratory-panel. 2020. Accessed June 23, 2021.

42. GenMark Dx. EPlex SARS-CoV-2 Test Assay Manual. Available at: https://www.fda.gov/media/136282/download. 2020. Accessed June 28, 2021.

43. GenMark Dx. EPlex Respiratory Pathogen Panel 2 Package Insert. Available at: https://www.fda.gov/media/142905/download. 2020. Accessed June 28, 2021.

44. Cepheid. Xpert Xpress SARS-CoV-2/Flu/RSV Instructions For Use. Available at: https://www.cepheid.com/en/package-inserts/1913. 2021. Accessed June 28, 2021.

45. Fournier PE, Zandotti C, Ninove L, et al. Contribution of VitaPCR SARS-CoV-2 to the emergency diagnosis of COVID-19. J Clin Virol 2020;133(January):337–9.

46. Qiagen. QIAstat-Dx Respiratory Panel. Instructions for Use. Available at: https://www.qiagen.com/us/resources/download.aspx?id=e3f2dc10-c712-4bcf-9acd-211bd35df944&lang=en. 2020. Accessed June 28, 2021.

47. Cepheid. Xpert Xpress SARS-CoV-2 Instructions For Use. Available at: https://www.cepheid.com/en/package-inserts/1615. 2020. Accessed June 28, 2021.

48. Lee J, Song JU. Diagnostic accuracy of the Cepheid Xpert Xpress and the Abbott ID NOW assay for rapid detection of SARS-CoV-2: a systematic review and meta-analysis. J Med Virol 2021;(March):1–9.

49. Fitoussi F, Dupont R, Tonen-Wolyec S, et al. Performances of the VitaPCR™ SARS-CoV-2 Assay during the second wave of the COVID-19 epidemic in France. J Med Virol 2021;(March):1–7.

50. Eckbo EJ, Locher K, Caza M, et al. Evaluation of the BioFire COVID-19 test and Respiratory Panel 2.1 for rapid identification of SARS-CoV-2 in nasopharyngeal swab samples. Diagn Microbiol Infect Dis 2021;99(3):115260.

51. Creager HM, Cabrera B, Schnaubelt A, et al. Clinical evaluation of the BioFire® Respiratory Panel 2.1 and detection of SARS-CoV-2. J Clin Virol 2020 Aug;129:104538. https://doi.org/10.1016/j.jcv.2020.104538.

52. Visseaux B, Le Hingrat Q, Collin G, et al. Evaluation of the QIAstat-dx respiratory SARS-CoV-2 Panel, the first rapid multiplex PCR commercial assay for SARS-CoV- 2 detection. J Clin Microbiol 2020;58(8):1–5.

53. Luminex. ARIES SARS-CoV-2 Assay Package Insert. Available at: https://www.fda.gov/media/136693/download. 2020. Accessed June 28, 2021.

54. MobiDiag. Novodiag COVID-19 Instructions For Use. Document Version 6-0. 2020.

55. Magleby R, Westblade LF, Trzebucki A, et al. Impact of severe acute respiratory syndrome Coronavirus 2 Viral load on risk of intubation and mortality among hospitalized patients with coronavirus disease 2019. Clin Infect Dis 2020.

56. Visseaux B, Le Q, Collin G, et al. Evaluation of the RealStar® SARS-CoV-2 RT-PCR kit RUO performances and limit of detection. J Clin Virol 2020;129:104520.

57. Public Health England. Rapid Assessment of the genetic signatures Easy-Screen SARS -CoV-2 detection kit. Available at: https://www.gov.uk/government/publications/covid-19-phe-laboratory-assessments-of-molecular-tests. 2020. Accessed June 23, 2021.

58. Freire-Paspuel B, Garcia-Bereguiain MA. Analytical sensitivity and clinical performance of a triplex RT-qPCR assay using CDC N1, N2, and RP targets for SARS-CoV-2 diagnosis. Int J Infect Dis 2021;102:14–6.

59. Kenyeres B, Anosi N, Banyai K, et al. Comparison of four PCR and two point of care assays used in the laboratory detection of SARS-CoV-2. J Virol Methods 2021;293.

60. Görzer I, Buchta C, Chiba P, et al. First results of a national external quality assessment scheme for the detection of SARS-CoV-2 genome sequences. J Clin Virol 2020;129. https://doi.org/10.1016/j.jcv.2020.104537.

61. Labbé AC, Benoit P, Gobeille Paré S, et al. Comparison of saliva with oral and nasopharyngeal swabs for SARS-CoV-2 detection on various commercial and laboratory-developed assays. J Med Virol 2021;1–6. https://doi.org/10.1002/jmv.27026.

62. Garg A, Ghoshal U, Patel SS, et al. Evaluation of seven commercial RT-PCR kits for COVID-19 testing in pooled clinical specimens. J Med Virol 2021;93(4):2281–6.

63. Price TK, Bowland BC, Chandrasekaran S, et al. Performance characteristics of severe acute respiratory syndrome coronavirus 2 RT-PCR tests in a single health system. J Mol Diagn 2021;23(2):159–63.

64. Cuong HQ, Hai ND, Linh HT, et al. Comparison of primer-probe sets among different master mixes for laboratory screening of severe acute respiratory syndrome Coronavirus 2 (SARS-CoV-2). Biomed Res Int 2020;2020. https://doi.org/10.1155/2020/7610678.

65. Procop GW, Brock JE, Reineks EZ, et al. A comparison of five SARS-CoV-2 molecular assays with clinical correlations. Am J Clin Pathol 2021;155(1):69–78.

66. Wirden M, Feghoul L, Bertine M, et al. Multicenter comparison of the Cobas 6800 system with the RealStar RT-PCR kit for the detection of SARS-CoV-2. J Clin Virol 2020;130.

67. Kohmer N, Rabenau HF, Hoehl S, et al. Comparative analysis of point-of-care, high-throughput and laboratory-developed SARS-CoV-2 nucleic acid amplification tests (NATs). J Virol Methods 2021;291. https://doi.org/10.1016/j.jviromet.2021.114102.

68. Lee CK, Tham JWM, Png S, et al. Clinical performance of Roche xobas 6800, Luminex ARIES, MiRXES fortitude kit 2.1, altona RealStar, and applied Biosystems TaqPath for SARS-CoV-2 detection in nasopharyngeal swabs. J Med Virol 2021;1–5. https://doi.org/10.1002/jmv.26940.

69. van Kasteren PB, van der Veer B, van den Brink S, et al. Comparison of seven commercial RT-PCR diagnostic kits for COVID-19. J Clin Virol 2020;128.

70. Merindol N, Pépin G, Marchand C, et al. SARS-CoV-2 detection by direct rRT-PCR without RNA extraction. J Clin Virol 2020;128:3–6.

71. Schnuriger A, Perrier M, Marinho V, et al. Caution in interpretation of SARS-CoV-2 quantification based on RT-PCR cycle threshold value. Diagn Microbiol Infect Dis 2021;100(3):2–5. https://doi.org/10.1016/j.diagmicrobio.2021.115366.

72. Public Health England. Rapid assessment of biomerieux real-time detection kit. Available at: https://www.gov.uk/government/publications/covid-19-phe-laboratory-assessments-of-molecular-tests. 2020. Accessed June 23, 2021.

73. Tastanova A, Stoffel CI, Dzung A, et al. A comparative study of real-time RT-PCR–based SARS-CoV-2 detection methods and its application to human-derived and surface swabbed material. J Mol Diagn 2021;23(7):796–804.

74. A.Menarini Diagnostics. CORONAMELT; 2020. Available at: https://www.menarinidiagnostics.com/en-us/Home/Laboratory-products/COVID-19/Viral-RNA-Detection/CoronaMelt/Overview. Accessed June 28, 2021.

75. Altona Diagnostics. The altona Diagnostics product portfolio. 2021. Available at: https://altona-diagnostics.com/en/the-altona-product-lines.html. Accessed June 28, 2021.
76. CerTest BioTec. VIASURE real time PCR detection kits SARS-CoV-2, FLU & RSV. Available at: https://www.certest.es/products/sars-cov-2-flu-rsv/, 2021. Accessed June 28, 2021.
77. Thermo Fisher scientific. TaqManTM SARS-CoV-2, Flu A/B, RSV RT-PCR assay kit. 2021. Available at: https://www.thermofisher.com/order/catalog/product/A47702#/A47702https://www.thermofisher.com/order/catalog/product/A47702#/A47702. Accessed June 28, 2021.
78. Vela diagnostics. ViroKey SARS-CoV-2 RT-PCR test v2.0 (CE-IVD). 2021. Available at. https://www.veladx.com/product/qpcr-respiratory-infections/virokey-sars-cov-2-rt-pcr-test-v20-ce-ivd.html. Accessed June 29, 2021.
79. Lima A, Healer V, Vendrone E, et al. Validation of a modified CDC assay and performance comparison with the NeuMoDxTM and DiaSorin® automated assays for rapid detection of SARS-CoV-2 in respiratory specimens. J Clin Virol 2020 Dec;133:104688. https://doi.org/10.1016/j.jcv.2020.104688.
80. Navarathna DH, Sharp S, Lukey J, et al. Understanding false positives and the detection of SARS-CoV-2 using the Cepheid Xpert Xpress SARS-CoV-2 and BD MAX SARS-CoV-2 assays. Diagn Microbiol Infect Dis 2021;100(1). https://doi.org/10.1016/j.diagmicrobio.2021.115334.
81. EliTech Group. SARS-CoV-2 PLUS ELITe MGB kit. 2020. Available at. https://www.elitechgroup.com/product/sars-cov-2-plus-elite-mgb-kit. Accessed June 28, 2021.
82. Aus Diagnostics. SARS-COV-2, INFLUENZA AND RSV 8-WELL Instructions for Use. 2021.
83. Mannonen L, Kallio-Kokko H, Loginov R, et al. Comparison of two commercial platforms and a laboratory-developed test for detection of severe acute respiratory syndrome Coronavirus 2 (SARS-CoV-2) RNA. J Mol Diagn 2021;23(4):407–16.
84. Mostafa HH, Hardick J, Morehead E, et al. Comparison of the analytical sensitivity of seven commonly used commercial SARS-CoV-2 automated molecular assays. J Clin Virol 2020;130. https://doi.org/10.1016/j.jcv.2020.104578.
85. Aretzweiler G, Leuchter S, Simon CO, et al. Generating timely molecular diagnostic test results: workflow comparison of the cobas® 6800/8800 to Panther. Expert Rev Mol Diagn 2019;19(10):951–7.
86. Khan KA, Cheung P. Presence of mismatches between diagnostic PCR assays and coronavirus SARS-CoV-2 genome: sequence mismatches in SARS-CoV-2 PCR. R Soc Open Sci 2020;7(6):200636.
87. Craney AR, Velu PD, Satlin MJ, et al. Comparison of two high-throughput reverse transcription-PCR systems for the detection of severe acute respiratory syndrome coronavirus 2. J Clin Microbiol 2020;58(8):1–6.
88. Lieberman J, Pepper G, Naccache S, et al. Comparison of commercially available and laboratory developed assays for in vitro detection of SARS-CoV-2 in clinical laboratories. J Clin Microbiol 2020;58(8):e00821-20.
89. Kogoj R, Kmetič P, Valenčak AO, et al. Real-life head-to-head comparison of performance of two high-throughput automated assays for detection of SARS-CoV-2 RNA in nasopharyngeal swabs: the Alinity m SARS-CoV-2 and cobas 6800 SARS-CoV-2 assays. J Mol Diagn 2021. https://doi.org/10.1016/j.jmoldx.2021.05.003.

90. Perchetti GA, Pepper G, Shrestha L, et al. Performance characteristics of the Abbott Alinity m SARS-CoV-2 assay. J Clin Virol 2021;140(May):104869.

91. Smith E, Zhen W, Manji R, et al. Analytical and clinical comparison of three nucleic acid amplification tests for SARS-CoV-2 detection. J Clin Microbiol 2020; 58(9):e01134-20.

92. Fung B, Gopez A, Servellita V, et al. Direct comparison of SARS-CoV-2 analytical limits of detection across seven molecular assays. J Clin Microbiol 2020;58(9): e01535-20.

93. Baker RE, Park SW, Yang W, et al. The impact of COVID-19 nonpharmaceutical interventions on the future dynamics of endemic infections. Proc Natl Acad Sci U S A 2020;117(48):30547–53.

94. Cheng A, Riedel S, Arnaout R, et al. Verification of the Abbott Alinity m Resp-4-Plex Assay for detection of SARS-CoV-2, influenza A/B, and respiratory syncytial virus. medRxiv 2021.

95. Cepheid. GeneXpert-Infinity. 2021. Available at: https://www.cepheid.com/en_US/systems/GeneXpert-Family-of-Systems/GeneXpert-Infinity. Accessed July 1, 2021.

96. Shahhosseini N, Babuadze G, Wong G, et al. Mutation signatures and in silico docking of novel sars-cov-2 variants of concern. Microorganisms 2021;9(5): 1–15. https://doi.org/10.3390/microorganisms9050926.

97. Davies NG, Abbott S, Barnard R, et al. Estimated transmissibility and impact of SARS-CoV-2 lineage B.1.1.7 in England. Science 2021;372(6538).

98. Tegally H, Wilkinson E, Giovanetti M, et al. Emergence and rapid spread of a new severe acute respiratory syndrome-related coronavirus 2 (SARS-CoV-2) lineage with multiple spike mutations in South Africa. medRxiv 2020;2. https://doi.org/10.1101/2020.12.21.20248640.

99. Andreano E, Piccini G, Licastro D, et al. SARS-CoV-2 escape in vitro from a highly neutralizing COVID-19 convalescent plasma. bioRxiv 2020. https://doi.org/10.1101/2020.12.28.424451.

100. Greaney AJ, Loes AN, Crawford KHD, et al. Comprehensive mapping of mutations in the SARS-CoV-2 receptor-binding domain that affect recognition by polyclonal human plasma antibodies. Cell Host Microbe 2021;29(3):463–76.e6.

101. Ramanathan K, Antognini D, Combes A, et al. Comprehensive mapping of mutations in the SARS CoV- 2 receptor-binding domain that affect recognition by polyclonal human plasma antibodies. Cell Host Microbe 2020;(January):19–21.

102. Weisblum Y, Schmidt F, Zhang F, et al. Escape from neutralizing antibodies 1 by SARS-CoV-2 spike protein variants. Elife 2020;9:1.

103. Rambaut A, Loman N, Pybus O, et al. Preliminary genomic characterisation of an emergent SARS-CoV-2 lineage in the UK defined by a novel set of spike mutations. Available at: https://virological.org/t/preliminary-genomic-characterisation-of-an-emergent-sars-cov-2-lineage-in-the-uk-defined-by-a-novel-set-of-spike-mutations/563. 2021. Accessed June 23, 2021.

104. Sabino EC, Buss LF, Carvalho MPS, et al. Resurgence of COVID-19 in Manaus, Brazil, despite high seroprevalence. Lancet 2021;397(10273):452–5.

105. Yi C, Sun X, Ye J, et al. Key residues of the receptor binding motif in the spike protein of SARS-CoV-2 that interact with ACE2 and neutralizing antibodies. Cell Mol Immunol 2020;17(6):621–30.

106. Cagliani R, Forni D, Clerici M, et al. Computational inference of selection underlying the evolution of the novel coronavirus, severe acute respiratory syndrome coronavirus 2. J Virol 2020;94(12):e00411-20.

107. Ou J, Zhou Z, Dai R, et al. Emergence of rbd mutations in circulating sars-cov-2 strains enhancing the structural stability and human ace2 receptor affinity of the spike protein. bioRxiv 2020;1–30.

108. World Health Organization. Tracking SARS-CoV-2 variants. 2021. Available at: https://www.who.int/en/activities/tracking-SARS-CoV-2-variants/. Accessed June 28, 2021.

109. Thermo Fisher scientific. TaqMan SARS-CoV-2 mutation Panel. 2021. Available at: https://www.thermofisher.com/uk/en/home/clinical/clinical-genomics/pathogen-detection-solutions/real-time-pcr-research-solutions-sars-cov-2/mutation-panel.html. Accessed June 29, 2021.

110. Bioscience A. MassARRAY® SARS-CoV-2 variant Panel (RUO). 2021. Available at: https://www.agenabio.com/wp-content/uploads/2021/03/GEN0048-05-SC2-Variant-Product-Sheet.pdf. Accessed July 1, 2021.

111. Kakhki RK, Kakhki MK, Neshani A. COVID-19 target: a specific target for novel coronavirus detection. Gene Rep 2020;20:100740.

112. Wu D, Koganti R, Lambe UP, et al. Vaccines and therapies in development for SARS-CoV-2 infections. J Clin Med 2020;9(6):1885.

113. Kim C-H. SARS-CoV-2 evolutionary adaptation toward host entry and recognition of receptor O-acetyl sialylation in virus–host interaction. Int J Mol Sci 2020;21(12):4549.

114. Huang C, Lokugamage KG, Rozovics JM, et al. SARS coronavirus nsp1 protein induces template-dependent endonucleolytic cleavage of mRNAs: viral mRNAs are resistant to nsp1-induced RNA cleavage. PLOS Pathog 2011;7(12):e1002433.

115. Cornillez-Ty CT, Liao L, Yates JR 3rd, et al. Severe acute respiratory syndrome coronavirus nonstructural protein 2 interacts with a host protein complex involved in mitochondrial biogenesis and intracellular signaling. J Virol 2009;83(19):10314–8.

116. Korber B, Fischer WM, Gnanakaran S, et al. Tracking changes in SARS-CoV-2 spike: evidence that D614G increases infectivity of the COVID-19 virus. Cell 2020;182(4):812–27.e19.

117. Oostra M, Te Lintelo EG, Deijs M, et al. Localization and membrane topology of coronavirus nonstructural protein 4: involvement of the early secretory pathway in replication. J Virol 2007;81(22):12323–36.

118. Chan JF-W, Kok K-H, Zhu Z, et al. Genomic characterization of the 2019 novel human-pathogenic coronavirus isolated from a patient with atypical pneumonia after visiting Wuhan. Emerg Microbes Infect 2020;9(1):221–36.

119. Benvenuto D, Angeletti S, Giovanetti M, et al. Evolutionary analysis of SARS-CoV-2: how mutation of Non-Structural Protein 6 (NSP6) could affect viral autophagy. J Infect 2020;81(1):e24–7.

120. Cottam EM, Whelband MC, Wileman T. Coronavirus NSP6 restricts autophagosome expansion. Autophagy 2014;10(8):1426–41.

121. Wang Y, Sun Y, Wu A, et al. Coronavirus nsp10/nsp16 methyltransferase can Be targeted by nsp10-derived peptide in vitro and in vivo to reduce replication and pathogenesis. J Virol 2015;89(16):8416–27.

122. Suryawanshi RK, Koganti R, Agelidis A, et al. Dysregulation of cell signaling by SARS-CoV-2. Trends Microbiol 2021;29(3):224–37.

123. Wu F, Zhao S, Yu B, et al. A new coronavirus associated with human respiratory disease in China. Nature 2020;579(7798):265–9.

124. Seybert A, Hegyi A, Siddell SG, et al. The human coronavirus 229E superfamily 1 helicase has RNA and DNA duplex-unwinding activities with 5'-to-3' polarity. Rna 2000;6(7):1056–68.

125. Chang C-k, Hou M-H, Chang C-F, et al. The SARS coronavirus nucleocapsid protein – forms and functions. Antiviral Res 2014;103:39–50.

126. Chen Y, Cai H, Pan J, et al. Functional screen reveals SARS coronavirus nonstructural protein nsp14 as a novel cap N7 methyltransferase. Proc Natl Acad Sci 2009;106(9):3484.

127. Naqvi AAT, Fatima K, Mohammad T, et al. Insights into SARS-CoV-2 genome, structure, evolution, pathogenesis and therapies: structural genomics approach. Biochim Biophys Acta Mol Basis Dis 2020;1866(10):165878.

128. Castaño-Rodriguez C, Honrubia JM, Gutiérrez-Álvarez J, et al. Role of severe acute respiratory syndrome coronavirus viroporins E, 3a, and 8a in replication and pathogenesis. mBio 2018;9(3):e02325-17.

129. Yount B, Roberts RS, Sims AC, et al. Severe acute respiratory syndrome coronavirus group-specific open reading frames encode nonessential functions for replication in cell cultures and mice. J Virol 2005;79(23):14909–22.

130. Xia H, Cao Z, Xie X, et al. Evasion of type I interferon by SARS-CoV-2. Cell Rep 2020;33(1):108234.

131. Chen S, Zheng X, Zhu J, et al. Extended ORF8 gene region is valuable in the epidemiological investigation of severe acute respiratory syndrome–similar coronavirus. J Infect Dis 2020;222(2):223–33.

132. Wang M-Y, Zhao R, Gao L-J, et al. SARS-CoV-2: structure, biology, and structure-based therapeutics development. Front Cell Infect Microbiol 2020; 10:724.

133. MobiDiag. Coronavirus solutions. 2021. Available at: https://mobidiag.com/products/coronavirus/. Accessed June 29, 2021.

134. MobiDiag. Amplidiag COVID-19 Instructions for Use. 2020.

135. Jokela P, Jääskeläinen AE, Jarva H, et al. SARS-CoV-2 sample-to-answer nucleic acid testing in a tertiary care emergency department: evaluation and utility. J Clin Virol 2020;131(January). https://doi.org/10.1016/j.jcv.2020.104614.

136. Aus diagnostics. Highplex Alliance™. 2021. Available at: https://www.ausdiagnostics.com/highplex-alliance. Accessed June 29, 2021.

137. Pham J, Meyer S, Nguyen C, et al. Performance characteristics of a high-throughput automated. J Clin Microbiol 2020;1–6.

138. Schneider M, Iftner T, Ganzenmueller T. Evaluation of the analytical performance and specificity of a SARS-CoV-2 transcription-mediated amplification assay. J Virol Methods 2021;294:114182.

139. Zhen W, Manji R, Smith E, et al. Comparison of four molecular in vitro diagnostic assays for the detection of sars-cov-2 in nasopharyngeal specimens. J Clin Microbiol 2020;58.

140. Wong RCW, Wong AH, Ho YII, et al. Performance evaluation of Panther Fusion SARS-CoV-2 assay for detection of SARS-CoV-2 from deep throat saliva, nasopharyngeal, and lower-respiratory-tract specimens. J Med Virol 2021;93: 1226–8.

141. Dust K, Hedley A, Nichol K, et al. Comparison of commercial assays and laboratory developed tests for detection of SARS-CoV-2. J Virol Methods 2020;285.

142. EliTech Group. SARS-CoV-2 variants ELITe MGB® kit. Available at: https://www.elitechgroup.com/product/sars-cov-2-variants-elite-mgb-kit. Accessed June 29, 2021.

143. CerTest BioTec. SARS-CoV-2 & UK variant (S UK, ORF1ab and N genes). 2021. Available at: https://www.certest.es/products/sars-cov-2-uk-variant-s-uk-orf1ab-and-n-genes/. Accessed June 29, 2021.
144. Antolia geneworks. Bosphore SARS-CoV-2 variant detection kit v1. 2021. Available at: http://www.anatoliageneworks.com/en/kitler.asp?id=375&baslik=Bosphore SARS-CoV-2 Variant Detection Kit v1&bas=Bosphore SARS-CoV-2 Variant Detection Kit v1. Accessed June 29, 2021.
145. TIB MOLBIOL. SARS kits and VirSNiP assays. 2021. Available at: https://www.tib-molbiol.de/covid-19. Accessed June 29, 2021.

SARS-CoV-2 Molecular Diagnostics in China

Yanjun Lu, PhD, Ziyong Sun, PhD*

KEYWORDS

- SARS-CoV-2 • Molecular diagnosis • Real-time PCR • Serologic assays

KEY POINTS

- Primers designed to target various RNA sequences within different genes of SARS-CoV-2 affect the sensitivity.
- Molecular techniques and serological assays widely used in China have the advantages and disadvantages of these techniques.
- Immunoassays have been developed for detection of COVID-19 but still as a complementary identification assay.

INTRODUCTION

Since the outbreak of coronavirus disease 2019 (COVID-19), the number of infected people has been increasing rapidly worldwide.[1,2] As of February 22, 2022, more than 420 million confirmed cases of COVID-19 and over 5.8 million deaths worldwide had been reported.[3] With effective prevention and control strategies, China won a significant early victory against COVID-19, and now mainly focuses on preventing the transmission of imported COVID-19.[4] One of the successful strategies in China is rapid and extensive detection of Severe Acute Respiratory Syndrome Coronavirus 2 (SARS-CoV-2) to decrease the risk of transmission by rapidly enabling isolation and contact tracing.

SARS-CoV-2 is a positive-sense, single-stranded RNA virus, and the whole viral genome is approximately 29,903 nt (GenBank, MN908947.3) in length.[5,6] SARS-CoV-2 consists of at least 12 coding regions, including open reading frames (ORF) 1 ab, S, 3, E, M, 7, 8, 9, 10b, N, 13, and 14.[6,7] Orf1ab and orf1a genes are located at the 5′-end of the genome, which encode pp1ab and pp1a proteins, respectively. The 3′-end of the genome encodes 4 structural proteins including spike, envelope, membrane, and nucleocapsid proteins, as well as accessory proteins. Genomic sequencing revealed that SARS-CoV-2 was closely related to bat-SL-CoVZC45 and

Department of Laboratory Medicine, Tongji Hospital, Tongji Medical College, Huazhong University of Science and Technology, Wuhan 430030, China
* Corresponding author.
E-mail address: zysun@tjh.tjmu.edu.cn

Clin Lab Med 42 (2022) 193–201
https://doi.org/10.1016/j.cll.2022.03.003
0272-2712/22/© 2022 Elsevier Inc. All rights reserved.

bat-CoV RaTG13 with a similarity of 88% and 96.3%, respectively,[8,9] whereas only shared about 79% and 50% sequences with SARS-CoV and MERS-CoV.[10]

According to Diagnosis & Treatment Scheme for Coronavirus Disease 2019 (7th Edition) in China, 3 methods have been used for the diagnosis of SARS-CoV-2 infection, including detection of positive SARS-CoV-2 nucleic acids by reverse transcription–polymerase chain reaction (RT-PCR), viral gene sequencing to detect known SARS-CoV-2 sequences, and the identification of positive SARS-CoV-2–specific IgM and IgG antibodies in serum.[11] Numerous commercial kits for SARS-CoV-2 have been developed and used in the battle against COVID-19. As of November 20, 2020, a total of 51 approved kits for SARS-CoV-2 had been approved by the National Medical Products Administration of China (NMPA), including 24 that detect nucleic acids (), 25 kits that detect antibodies , and 2 kits targeting antigens .[12] High-throughput sequencing, RT-PCR, RT-loop–mediated isothermal amplification (RT-LAMP) have been widely used for SARS-CoV-2 nucleic acid detection,[13–15] and RT-PCR is recommended in the guideline for the COVID-19 diagnosis and treatment program in China.[16] The serologic assays mainly include lateral flow immunoassay (LFIA), chemiluminescence immunoassay (CLIA), or enzyme-linked immunosorbent assay (ELISA), used to detect antibodies produced by individuals exposed to SARS-CoV-2. Some LFIA-based antigen detection kits have been developed recently.

This review summarizes the molecular techniques and serologic assays widely used in China and discusses the advantages and disadvantages of these techniques. In brief, it is crucial to select appropriate diagnostic methods or combine different methods and other clinical parameters to confirm the SARS-CoV-2 infection status of individuals.

REVERSE TRANSCRIPTION—POLYMERASE CHAIN REACTION

Nucleic acid detection is an important diagnostic tool for the clinical diagnosis, segregation, rehabilitation, and discharge of patients, and was also applied as the "gold standard" for the detection of SARS-CoV-2 infection in the early stage of the epidemic. Currently, numerous primers are designed to target various RNA sequences within 6 genes of SARS-CoV-2 including ORF1a/b, ORF1b-nsp14 (50-UTR), RdRp (RNA-dependent RNA polymerase), S, E, N1/N2/N3, and RdRp/Hel (RNA-dependent RNA polymerase/helicase).[17] The Chinese Center for Disease Control and Prevention (CDC) recommends the use of primers and fluorescent probes targeting SARS-CoV-2 ORF1ab and nucleocapsid protein (N) gene regions.[18] The CDC in America recommends two nucleocapsid targets (N1, N2,), whereas Europe recommends initial screening with E gene followed by confirmation targeting the RdRp.[19,20] SARS-CoV-2 has low homology with other bat-related viruses in the ORF1b (involving RdRp), N, and S genes, which are relatively specific genes worth targeting.[21,22] Recent clinical evaluations have further demonstrated that the N1, N2, and E gene detection assays have better performance than the RdRP and N3 detection assays.[23] More recently, Chan and colleagues designed novel primers and probes for real-time RT-PCR detection of RdRp/Helicase (Hel), S and N genes, which was more sensitive than assays targeting other genes.[24]

At the start of the epidemic in China, RT-PCR kits were developed rapidly and had the earliest clinical application; however, the sensitivity of RT-PCR results was only 30% to 50%.[25] This is due to a variety of factors, including low viral loads in specimens such as throat swabs and other respiratory samples, samples not being properly preserved, and the technology itself, which would be affected by virus mutation and PCR inhibitor.[25,26] Viral loads of respiratory tract specimens are highest in bronchoalveolar lavage fluid(BALF), followed by sputum, nasal swabs, and pharyngeal swabs;

however, in clinical application, nasopharyngeal and oropharyngeal swabs served as the main sample types for clinical testing due to ease of sampling . Because of the limited sensitivity of RT-PCR, a negative results from an oral-nasopharyngeal swab was not sufficient for hospital discharge in China.[27,28] Virus inactivation before testing should also be considered to cause false-negative results. Thermal inactivation of samples at 56°C for 30 min was recommended to ensure biosafety for laboratory personnel before SARS-CoV-2 RNA detection.[29] However, approximately half of the weakly positive samples were RT-PCR negative after thermal inactivation of SARS-CoV-2 at 56°C for 45 min in parallel testing.[30]

A series of assays have been approved by the NMPA with Emergency Use Authorization in response to COVID-19 infection; however, the analytical performance claimed in the corresponding instructions by manufacturers has not been thoroughly validated. In clinical applications, the differences in nucleic acid extraction methods, RT-PCR processes, personnel, or equipment lead to variations in testing results among different laboratories.[31] Nucleic acid extraction is one of the most critical steps for nucleic acid detection to ensure the reliability of molecular diagnosis.[32] In China, various nucleic acid extraction methods were applied by the laboratories. Among these methods, manual column-based, manual magnetic bead-based, automated column-based, and automated magnetic bead-based methods accounted for 21.3% (198/931), 15.3% (142/931), 1.5% (14/931), and 51.7% (481/931), respectively.[33] For each positive sample of external quality assessment, the percentage agreement of the laboratories using magnetic bead-based extraction method was higher than those using column-based extraction method.[33]

False-negative results could potentially arise from mutations occurring in the primer and probe-target regions in the SARS-CoV-2 genome.[34] As RNA viruses have a high degree of genetic variability, mismatches between primers and target sequences caused by mutations can lead to poor detection performance. The results should be validated with different primer sets against the same gene and combined with patient history and other clinical data to accurately determine SARS-CoV-2 infection status.[35]

HIGH-THROUGHPUT SEQUENCING

In the early stage of the epidemic, the metagenomics next-generation sequencing (mNGS) was used to identify and analyze the genome of SARS-CoV-2 within 5 days by the Chinese CDC. The phylogenetic analysis of these genomes showed that the similarity between the genomic sequence of SARS-CoV-2 and SARS or bat-derived strains were 79% and 88%, respectively.[6] The first mNGS system related to the ultra-high-throughput sequencer DNBSEQ-T7, with the supporting analysis software and nucleic acid detection kits, has been approved by the NMPA, which can identify and diagnose coronaviruses, including SARS-CoV-2 and other infectious respiratory pathogens, and enable rapid detection of viral sequences.[36] Nanopore sequencing is a third-generation genome sequencing technology providing real-time analysis and rapid insights, which does not require enzymes to amplify samples and directly performs full-length sequencing of SARS-CoV-2 and additional respiratory viruses within a few hours.[37,38] However, NGS is currently impractical for routine use in most clinical laboratories for the diagnosis of SARS-CoV-2 infection due to some limitations, such as the high cost and long testing cycles.

ISOTHERMAL AMPLIFICATION ASSAYS

Isothermal amplification of nucleic acid is a method for the rapid and efficient accumulation of nucleic acid at a specific constant temperature. RT-LAMP has been introduced to detect SARS-CoV-2 with a series of 4 target-specific primers targeting 6-different regions of the genome in a combined LAMP and reverse transcription-based methodology.[39] RT-LAMP showed a high degree of specificity (99.5%), sensitivity (91.4%) compared with RT-qPCR for identification of SARS-CoV-2.[40] Currently, point-of-care testing (POCT) of SARS-CoV-2 in nasal swabs using RT-LAMP from Abbott Diagnostics has been approved by US FDA. However, it is restricted to one sample per run.[41] Relevant products have been also approved by the NMPA in China as a potential POCT method in airports, community clinics, and hospitals. The limitations of RT-LAMP assays are that the technology is more complicated than RT-PCR and involves multiple pairs of primers, limiting the choice of target sites and resolution or specificity.[42]

CRISPR-BASED NEWLY DEVELOPED METHODS

The CRISPR/Cas is a gene-editing toolbox, a combination of guide RNA (CRISPR RNA or crRNA) and Cas enzyme complex for detecting various target sequences and being applied in diagnostic microbiology and biomedicine. Recently, CRISPR has been developed for the detection of SARS-Cov-2 in China and the clinical sensitivity and specificity are comparable to RT-qPCR.[43,44] Owing to yield rapid read-outs and sensitive results of CRISPR, which is suitable candidates for simple POCT when coupled with lateral flow readouts.

ANTIBODY DETECTION ASSAYS

Serologic IgM/IgG antibody detection is suggested as a complementary identification assay to indirectly confirm SARS-CoV-2 infection. Briefly, the detection of specific antibodies can provide serologic evidence for infection and help confirm the diagnosis in patients with negative nucleic acid tests but high clinical suspicion.[45] In SARS-CoV-2 infection, RBD, S, and N proteins serve as the main antigens to stimulate the immune response of the body, producing IgA, IgM, and IgG antibodies. Particularly, the S1 subunit was more specific than S2 in detecting the SARS-CoV-2-specific antibodies.[46] The seroconversion of specific IgM and IgG antibodies against SARS-CoV-2 typically turn positive in the second or third week after symptom onset, but IgA and IgM were both detectable at the 5th day (median), whereas IgG appeared on the 14th day (median) in another study.[47] It has been reported that IgM peaks around 15 to 21 days after infection then slowly began to decline, whereas IgG peaks at 22 to 39 days and lasts for a longer time.[48] IgM and IgG antibodies convert to negative around 36 days and over 50 days, respectively.[47]

Currently, immunoassays have been developed for the detection of COVID-19 infection in serum, plasma, and whole blood. Among these strategies, LFIAs based on gold particles, up-converting phosphor, or quantum dot fluorescence, along with CLIA and ELISA, are the most promising approaches. The LFIA is user-friendly, cheap, and easily mass-produced, and the main advantage of LFIA is its potential usage for POCT. The diagnostic performance of 7 IgG/IgM LFIA kits has been evaluated for detecting SARS-CoV-2 antibodies in COVID-19 patients, and the specificity was $\geq$ 90.3% for IgG, $\geq$ 91.3% for IgM, and $\geq$97.1% for the combination IgM and IgG. The sensitivity 14 to25 days after onset of symptoms of the IgG LFIA was $\geq$ 92.1%.[49] Another study has reported that the sensitivity of the NG-Test was estimated to be 85% (95% confidence interval [CI]71.9%-92.3%) and the specificity 98.3% (95% CI 95.0%-100.0%) for both IgG and IgM when compared with the ELISA Wantai Immunoassay.[50] Another meta-analysis reported the sensitivity/specificity of CLIA, ELISA, and LFIA were 92% (95% CI: 86%-95%)/99% (CI: 97%-99%), 86% (CI:

82%-89%)/99% (CI: 98%-100%), and 78% (CI: 71%-83%)/98% (95% CI: 96%-99%), respectively.[51] CLIA platforms are widely used as serologic techniques for the quantitative detection of specific antigens or antibodies, which are believed to be promising emerging methods for SARS-CoV-2 antibody detection.

Serologic testing also has some limitations. The slow antibody response to SARS-CoV-2 virus indicates that they cannot be helpful in the early stages of infection. Thus, serologic testing alone cannot be used for diagnosis or exclusion of SARS-CoV-2 infection. Furthermore, it is also not suitable for general population screening.[52] False-positive detection of IgM and IgG antibodies has been described, mainly associated with the manufacturer-determined cut-off values of the kit. A weak positive result near the cut-off value is likely to be a false positive.[53] Another reason for false-positive results is interfering substances in plasma samples including interferon, rheumatoid factors and nonspecific antibodies.[54] In addition, potential cross-reactivity of SARS-CoV-2 antibodies with antibodies generated by other coronaviruses could also results in false-positive results.[55]

ANTIGEN-BASED ASSAYS FOR SARS-CoV-2

Recently, 2 antigen-based kits for rapid SARS-CoV-2 detection have been approved by the NMPA of China. These antigen-based detection kits were developed based on LFIA using the double antibody sandwich method.[36] With RT-PCR assay as the reference standard, the sensitivity, specificity, and percentage agreement of nucleocapsid protein antigen testing by the fluorescence immunochromatographic assay was 75.6% (95% CI, 69.0–81.3), 100% (95% CI, 91.1–100), and 80.5% (95% CI, 75.1–84.9) respectively, suggesting high specificity and relatively high sensitivity in SARS-CoV-2 diagnosis in the early phase of infection.[56] Although antigen tests may detect virus early in infection, they may have lower sensitivity compared with nucleic acid amplification tests and may cross-react with other coronaviruses.[57]

SUMMARY

Although the application of mNGS technology played an important role in detecting the pathogen SARS-CoV-2 in the early stage of the epidemic in Wuhan, RT-PCR is still the gold standard for the diagnosis of COVID-19 and plays an essential role in patient management as well as infection control. POCT molecular testing platforms such as Qiagen's, BioFire's Filmarray and Cepheid's GeneXpert can deliver fast, safe, simple, and accurate molecular detection of pathogens such as COVID-19, which are believed to be promising emerging methods for SARS-CoV-2 detection.

SARS-CoV-2 has evolved during the past two years, and the viruses have displayed a large number of genetic variations. This may cause mismatches between primers, probes, and target sequences, and lead to reduced detection performance and false-negative results. To prevent this, RT-PCR primer sets should be updated according to the genetic variants in SARS-CoV-2 genomic sequences.

In the future, novel epidemics or pandemics may be inevitable. There are various types of pneumonia-related pathogens, including SARS-CoV-2, SARS-CoV, influenza virus, parainfluenza virus, adenovirus, respiratory syncytial virus, rhinovirus, mycoplasma, and Chlamydia. It is necessary to focus on the development of detection technologies and supporting reagents that can simultaneously rapidly detect dozens of pathogens, while still being the high-throughput and low-cost differential diagnostic technologies.

CLINICS CARE POINTS

- RT-PCR is recommended in the guidelines for the COVID-19 diagnosis and treatment program in China due to simple operation, high throughput screening and super sensitivity.
- Serological IgM/IgG antibody detection is suggested as a complementary identification assay to indirectly confirm SARS-CoV-2 infection due to detect not the pathogen itself and the slow antibody response.

REFERENCES

1. Zhu N, Zhang D, Wang W, et al. A novel coronavirus from patients with pneumonia in China, 2019. N Engl J Med 2020;382(8):727–33.
2. Wang C, Horby PW, Hayden FG, et al. A novel coronavirus outbreak of global health concern. Lancet 2020;395(10223):470–3.
3. World Health Organization. Coronavirus disease (COVID-19) outbreak situation. Available at. http://www.who.int/emergen cies/diseases/novel-coronavirus-2019. Accessed Feb 2022.
4. Li Z, Chen Q, Feng L, et al. Active case finding with case management: the key to tackling the COVID-19 pandemic. Lancet 2020;396(10243):63–70.
5. Chan JF, Kok KH, Zhu Z, et al. Genomic characterization of the 2019 novel human-pathogenic coronavirus isolated from a patient with atypical pneumonia after visiting Wuhan. Emerg Microbes Infect 2020;9(1):221–36.
6. Lu R, Zhao X, Li J, et al. Genomic characterisation and epidemiology of 2019 novel coronavirus: implications for virus origins and receptor binding. Lancet 2020;395(10224):565–74.
7. Wu A, Peng Y, Huang B, et al. Genome composition and divergence of the novel coronavirus (2019-nCoV) originating in China. Cell Host Microbe 2020;27(3):325–8.
8. Lu J, du Plessis L, Liu Z, et al. Genomic epidemiology of SARS-CoV-2 in guang-dong province, China. Cell 2020;181(5):997–1003 e1009.
9. Paraskevis D, Kostaki EG, Magiorkinis G, et al. Full-genome evolutionary analysis of the novel corona virus (2019-nCoV) rejects the hypothesis of emergence as a result of a recent recombination event. Infect Genet Evol 2020;79:104212.
10. Chen L, Liu W, Zhang Q, et al. RNA based mNGS approach identifies a novel human coronavirus from two individual pneumonia cases in 2019 Wuhan outbreak. Emerg Microbes Infect 2020;9(1):313–9.
11. Zhao JY, Yan JY, Qu JM. Interpretations of "diagnosis and treatment protocol for novel coronavirus pneumonia (trial version 7). Chin Med J (Engl) 2020;133(11):1347–9.
12. Ruhan A, Wang H, Wang W, et al. Summary of the detection kits for SARS-CoV-2 approved by the national medical products administration of China and their application for diagnosis of COVID-19. Virol Sin 2020;35(6):699–712.
13. Waggoner JJ, Stittleburg V, Pond R, et al. Triplex real-time RT-PCR for Severe acute respiratory syndrome coronavirus 2. Emerg Infect Dis 2020;26(7):1633–5.
14. Dao Thi VL, Herbst K, Boerner K, et al. A colorimetric RT-LAMP assay and LAMP-sequencing for detecting SARS-CoV-2 RNA in clinical samples. Sci Transl Med 2020;12(556).
15. Zenker S, Kock F. The coronavirus pandemic - a critical discussion of a tourism research agenda. Tour Manag 2020;81:104164.

16. General Office of National Health Commission of the People's Republic of China. Prevention and control scheme for novel coronavirus pneumonia (version 2) [Internet]. 2020. Available at. http://wwwnhcgovcn/jkj/s3577/202001/c67cfe29ecf1470e8c7fc47d3b751e88shtml.

17. Abduljalil JM. Laboratory diagnosis of SARS-CoV-2: available approaches and limitations. New Microbes New Infect 2020;36:100713.

18. National Institute for Viral Disease Control and Prevention. Chinese center for disease control and prevention: novel coronavirus national science and technology resource service system[EB/OL]. 2020. Available at. http://nmdccn/nCov/en.

19. The Food and Drug Administration. CDC 2019-novel coronavirus (2019-nCoV) real-time RT-PCR diagnostic panel. Available at. http://www.fda.gov/media/134922/download (Accessed March 2020).

20. Corman VM, Landt O, Kaiser M, et al. Detection of 2019 novel coronavirus (2019-nCoV) by real-time RT-PCR. Euro Surveill 2020;25(3).

21. Zhou P, Yang XL, Wang XG, et al. A pneumonia outbreak associated with a new coronavirus of probable bat origin. Nature 2020;579(7798):270–3.

22. Chu DKW, Pan Y, Cheng SMS, et al. Molecular diagnosis of a novel coronavirus (2019-nCoV) causing an outbreak of pneumonia. Clin Chem 2020;66(4):549–55.

23. Nalla AK, Casto AM, Huang MW, et al. Comparative performance of SARS-CoV-2 detection assays using seven different primer-probe sets and one assay kit. J Clin Microbiol 2020;58(6).

24. Chan JF, Yip CC, To KK, et al. Improved molecular diagnosis of COVID-19 by the novel, highly sensitive and specific COVID-19-RdRp/Hel real-time reverse transcription-PCR Assay validated in vitro and with clinical specimens. J Clin Microbiol 2020;58(5).

25. Li N, Wang P, Wang X, et al. Molecular diagnosis of COVID-19: current situation and trend in China (Review). Exp Ther Med 2020;20(5):13.

26. Ji T, Liu Z, Wang G, et al. Detection of COVID-19: a review of the current literature and future perspectives. Biosens Bioelectron 2020;166:112455.

27. Wang W, Xu Y, Gao R, et al. Detection of SARS-CoV-2 in different types of clinical specimens. JAMA 2020;323(18):1843–4.

28. Wang X, Tan L, Wang X, et al. Comparison of nasopharyngeal and oropharyngeal swabs for SARS-CoV-2 detection in 353 patients received tests with both specimens simultaneously. Int J Infect Dis 2020;94:107–9.

29. National Health Commission of the People's Republic of China. Technical guide for prevention and control of coronavirus disease 2019 in medical institutions. 5th edition 2020 (in Chinese)Available at. http://www.nhc.gov.cn/jkj/s3577/202002/a5d6f7b8c48c451c87dba14889b30147.shtml.

30. Pan Y, Long L, Zhang D, et al. Potential false-negative nucleic acid testing results for severe acute respiratory syndrome coronavirus 2 from thermal inactivation of samples with low viral loads. Clin Chem 2020;66(6):794–801.

31. Sung H, Han MG, Yoo CK, et al. Nationwide external quality assessment of SARS-CoV-2 molecular testing, South Korea. Emerg Infect Dis 2020;26(10):2353–60.

32. Ali N, Rampazzo RCP, Costa ADT, et al. Current nucleic acid extraction methods and their implications to point-of-care diagnostics. Biomed Res Int 2017;2017:9306564.

33. Wang Z, Chen Y, Yang J, et al. External quality assessment for molecular detection of severe acute respiratory syndrome coronavirus 2 (SARS-CoV-2) in clinical laboratories. J Mol Diagn 2021;23(1):19–28.

34. Tahamtan A, Ardebili A. Real-time RT-PCR in COVID-19 detection: issues affecting the results. Expert Rev Mol Diagn 2020;20(5):453–4.

35. Shen Z, Xiao Y, Kang L, et al. Genomic diversity of severe acute respiratory syndrome-coronavirus 2 in patients with coronavirus disease 2019. Clin Infect Dis 2020;71(15):713–20.

36. China National Medical Products Administration. Registration information of domestic new coronavirus detection reagents. Available at. http://www.nmpa.gov.cn/WS04/CL2582/. http://english.nmpa.gov.cn.

37. Li J, Wang H, Mao L, et al. Rapid genomic characterization of SARS-CoV-2 viruses from clinical specimens using nanopore sequencing. Sci Rep 2020; 10(1):17492.

38. Wang M, Fu A, Hu B, et al. Nanopore targeted sequencing for the accurate and comprehensive detection of SARS-CoV-2 and other respiratory viruses. Small 2020;16(32):e2002169.

39. Yan C, Cui J, Huang L, et al. Rapid and visual detection of 2019 novel coronavirus (SARS-CoV-2) by a reverse transcription loop-mediated isothermal amplification assay. Clin Microbiol Infect 2020;26(6):773–9.

40. Jiang M, Pan W, Arasthfer A, et al. Development and validation of a rapid, single-step reverse transcriptase loop-mediated isothermal amplification (RT-LAMP) system potentially to be used for reliable and high-throughput screening of COVID-19. Front Cell Infect Microbiol 2020;10:331.

41. Carter LJ, Garner LV, Smoot JW, et al. Assay techniques and test development for COVID-19 diagnosis. ACS Cent Sci 2020;6(5):591–605.

42. Li Y, Fan P, Zhou S, et al. Loop-mediated isothermal amplification (LAMP): a novel rapid detection platform for pathogens. Microb Pathog 2017;107:54–61.

43. Hou T, Zeng W, Yang M, et al. Development and evaluation of a rapid CRISPR-based diagnostic for COVID-19. PLoS Pathog 2020;16(8):e1008705.

44. Qiu F, Wang H, Zhang Z, et al. [Laboratory testing techniques for SARS-CoV-2]. Nan Fang Yi Ke Da Xue Xue Bao 2020;40(2):164–7.

45. Jacofsky D, Jacofsky EM, Jacofsky M. Understanding antibody testing for COVID-19. J Arthroplasty 2020;35(7S):S74–81.

46. Okba NMA, Muller MA, Li W, et al. Severe acute respiratory syndrome coronavirus 2-specific antibody responses in coronavirus disease patients. Emerg Infect Dis 2020;26(7):1478–88.

47. Guo L, Ren L, Yang S, et al. Profiling early humoral response to diagnose novel coronavirus disease (COVID-19). Clin Infect Dis 2020;71(15):778–85.

48. Wu LX, Wang H, Gou D, et al. Clinical significance of the serum IgM and IgG to SARS-CoV-2 in coronavirus disease-2019. J Clin Lab Anal 2021;35(1):e23649.

49. Van Elslande J, Houben E, Depypere M, et al. Diagnostic performance of seven rapid IgG/IgM antibody tests and the euroimmun IgA/IgG ELISA in COVID-19 patients. Clin Microbiol Infect 2020;26(8):1082–7.

50. Garlantezec R, Heslan C, Tadie E, et al. A lateral flow immunoassay test performance in SARS-CoV-2 seroprevalence surveys: a validation study among healthcare workers. Emerg Microbes Infect 2020;9(1):2547–9.

51. Mekonnen D, Mengist HM, Derbie A, et al. Diagnostic accuracy of serological tests and kinetics of severe acute respiratory syndrome coronavirus 2 antibody: a systematic review and meta-analysis. Rev Med Virol 2020;31(3):e2181.

52. General Offce of National Health Commission of the People's Republic of China. Prevention and control scheme for novel coronavirus pneumonia (version 2) [Internet]. 2020. Available at. http://wwwnhcgovcn/jkj/s3577/202001/c67cfe29ecf1470e8c7fc-3b751e88shtml.

53. Latiano A, Tavano F, Panza A, et al. False-positive results of SARS-CoV-2 IgM/IgG antibody tests in sera stored before the 2020 pandemic in Italy. Int J Infect Dis 2021;104:159–63.
54. Deeks JJ, Dinnes J, Takwoingi Y, et al. Antibody tests for identification of current and past infection with SARS-CoV-2. Cochrane Database Syst Rev 2020;6: CD013652.
55. Udugama B, Kadhiresan P, Kozlowski HN, et al. Diagnosing COVID-19: the disease and tools for detection. ACS Nano 2020;14(4):3822–35.
56. Diao B, Wen K, Zhang J, et al. Accuracy of a nucleocapsid protein antigen rapid test in the diagnosis of SARS-CoV-2 infection. Clin Microbiol Infect 2021;27(2): 289 e281–4.
57. European Centre for disease Prevention and Control. An overview of the rapid test situation for COVID-19 diagnosis in the EU/EEA. Stockholm: European Centre for disease Prevention and Control; 2020. https://www.ecdc.europa.eu/sites/default/files/documents/Overview-rapid-test-situation-for-COVID-19-diagnosis-EU-EEA.pdf.

Rapid Antigen Assays for SARS-CoV-2: Promise and Peril

Thao T. Truong, PhD[a], Jennifer Dien Bard, PhD[a,b],
Susan M. Butler-Wu, PhD[b,*]

KEYWORDS

- SARS-CoV-2 • COVID-19 • Rapid antigen testing

KEY POINTS

- Rapid antigen detection tests (RADTs) for SARS-CoV-2 are most likely to be positive when viral loads are higher.
- The diagnostic performance characteristics of RADTs vary widely among different test brands, patient populations, and symptomatic status.
- RADTs enable more widescale scaling-up of testing globally. However, they are not appropriate as a test to determine infectiousness.
- In practice, the use of antigen testing to screen asymptomatic persons appears to work best when combined with other public health measures and not as a sole intervention method.

INTRODUCTION

The emergence of severe acute respiratory syndrome coronavirus 2 (SARS-CoV-2) initially caught many countries on the backfoot. The trials and tribulations of the initial roll-out of coronavirus disease 2019 (COVID-19) testing in the United States are well documented.[1] Although the specifics are beyond the scope of this article, they were numerous and well-publicized: from unavailability of swabs, reagents, and pipette tips to regulatory hurdles, initial testing stumbled in the United States in the face of a global pandemic caused by a novel virus.

Although reverse transcription–polymerase chain reaction (RT-PCR) and transcription-mediated amplification (TMA, hereafter PCR) remain the gold standard for the detection of SARS-CoV-2, at the time of writing, such testing still remains predominantly confined to diagnostic laboratories.[2] In contrast, rapid antigen detection tests (RADTs) lend themselves to widespread deployment because of their relatively

[a] Department of Pathology and Laboratory Medicine, Children's Hospital Los Angeles, Los Angeles, CA, USA; [b] Department of Pathology, Keck School of Medicine of the University of Southern California, Los Angeles, CA, USA
* Corresponding author.
E-mail address: butlerwu@usc.edu

Clin Lab Med 42 (2022) 203–222
https://doi.org/10.1016/j.cll.2022.03.001
0272-2712/22/© 2022 Elsevier Inc. All rights reserved.

low cost, and in many cases, the ability to be run without the use of specialized equipment.[3] This makes testing possible for clinics, geographic areas without proximal access to laboratories, and even in one's own home. RADTs have the potential to relieve pressure on diagnostic laboratories, who even well into 2022, continue to face labor and supply chain constraints. They represent a chance at test scalability beyond what can reasonably be achieved by diagnostic laboratory-based testing models.

SARS-CoV-2 viral loads are similar between asymptomatic and symptomatic cases and it was recognized relatively early in the pandemic that asymptomatic individuals are an important epidemiologic driver of spread.[4] Infrequent recovery of SARS-CoV-2 in culture after the first week of symptoms in mild-to-moderate cases, as well as the relatively high correlation between positive antigen test results and viral culture, led to the perception that RADTs could serve a role in assessing the presence of infectious virus.[5,6] Antigen testing has been touted as key in "returning to normal," with the concept of knowing ones "infectiousness status" having been widely popularized. Nevertheless, this concept is not without controversy or scientific counter-argument. Here, we discuss the utility of SARS-CoV-2 antigen testing, the unique opportunities it presents, and important considerations surrounding its use.

BACKGROUND

Before the COVID-19 pandemic, RADTs for respiratory viruses were historically associated with suboptimal test performance. This was dramatically illustrated during the emergence of novel H1N1 influenza A, where sensitivities of RADTs were found to be as low as 17.8%.[7] Meta-analyses evaluating the performance of influenza RADTs showed pooled sensitivities of 64.6% (95% confidence interval [CI], 59.0%–70.1%) and 52.2% (95% CI, 45.0%–59.3%) for influenza A and B, respectively, with pooled specificities of 98.2% (95% CI, 97.5%–98.7%).[8] Subsequent refinements such as the use of digital readers led to tests with improved sensitivities of up to 80%,[9] nevertheless, RADTs for influenza are less sensitive than molecular methods, with the Centers for Disease Control and Prevention (CDC) recommending confirmatory testing of negative specimens when influenza infection is suspected.[10,11]

Important differences between SARS-CoV-2 and other respiratory viruses inform how we might think about the potential utility of antigen testing for COVID-19. Although asymptomatic transmission was initially thought to be responsible for more than half of all COVID-19 cases, more recent estimates range between 17% and 30%.[12] In contrast, rates of asymptomatic influenza transmission are much lower.[13] Interestingly, influenza viral loads are 1 to 2 log10 copies lower among asymptomatic individuals, which may account in part for these lower transmission rates, though other studies refute this.[14,15] To prevent transmission of SARS-CoV-2 in hospital settings, many facilities in the United States perform PCR before surgery or other procedures (eg, colonoscopy), and even upon hospital admission.[16,17] Such testing has thus further compounded test demand for SARS-CoV-2 in traditional diagnostic laboratory settings. Arguably never before in the history of laboratory medicine has there been such high diagnostic testing demand for one agent of infection. It is into this landscape that massive interest in antigen testing for COVID-19 has emerged.

"Can I HAVE 'What IS THE REFERENCE METHOD? FOR $800"?

PCR is widely recognized as the most sensitive method to diagnose respiratory viral infections, having almost entirely replaced other previously commonly used test methods (ie, viral culture, direct fluorescence, etc). Nevertheless, an unfortunate and erroneous perception has emerged among the general public that PCR lacks specificity for SARS-CoV-2 detection. This stems from observations of SARS-CoV-2 RNA detectability for extended periods, long after resolution of infection.[4] Cycle threshold (Ct) values are typically high (>35) in such cases (ie, generally above the assay's limit of detection [LoD]) and repeat testing in these cases, therefore, oscillates between detection and nondetection.[18] High Ct values themselves do not necessarily indicate resolved infection, as such values can also be observed early in the infection course (before an exponential increase in viral loads) as well as among patients admitted to hospital with symptomatic disease.[19] Importantly, analytical false-positive SARS-CoV-2 PCR results have been shown to occur extremely rarely, though issues with specific assays have been observed.[20–22]

RADTs detect viral protein, usually viral nucleocapsid in the case of SARS-CoV-2. Nasal and nasopharyngeal specimens are predominantly used, with throat and saliva performing poorly for several RADT brands.[23–25] Chemiluminescent antigen tests may be compatible across all sample types.[26] Although commonly referred to in the popular press as if they are monolithic, there are countless different antigen test brands available worldwide, with 45 having received emergency use authorization (EUA) by the US Food and Drug Administration (FDA) at the time of writing.[27] Critically, not all brands perform equivalently: of 64 different antigen tests directly compared in one seminal study, only 29% met minimum performance standards defined as $\geq$97% sensitivity and an LoD of 60% at 100 plaque-forming units per milliliter.[28,29]

Regardless of the brand tested, some common principles have emerged: (1) SARS-CoV-2 RADTs are more likely to be positive when viral loads are higher, and (2) they are less likely to be positive after the first week of symptoms. High rates of antigen positivity are generally observed when Ct values are lower (ie, higher quantities of viral RNA detected), and when it is still possible to isolate infectious (ie, replication-competent) viruses in vitro.[30] For example, although sensitivity of the Innova assay was 78.2% overall in one study, sensitivity was 97% for specimens with Ct values < 25, and 95.5% for Ct values less than 28.[31] Similar findings have been observed for many assays across a multitude of studies.[28,32] It is important to recognize that Ct values vary widely and differ enormously between assays and laboratories.[33] Furthermore, Ct values are dramatically impacted by specimen quality and can be artificially high for poor-quality specimens, with poor specimen collection contributing to falsely negative results.[34]

Detection of culturable virus peaks near the time of symptom onset, with the probability of isolating infectious virus reduced to 6% after 10 days of symptoms among patients with mild-moderate infection.[35] Low rates of viral culture positivity have generally been observed for upper respiratory tract specimens with high Ct values,[35] but isolation of infectious virus has been observed for extended periods among patients with severe-to-critical illness[36] and among adults and children with prolonged severe immune compromise.[37,38] Although viral culturability is related to Ct value, cytopathic effects were observed among 43% of patients with severe infection and Ct values $\geq$ 26, compared with 22% for mild-to-moderate cases and even from specimens with Ct values $\geq$ 35 (5% in mild cases, 15% in severe cases).[39] Consequently, the relationship between high Ct values and the absence of culturability is not absolute; viral culturability can and does occur among specimens with high Ct values, albeit less frequently.

The high correlation between culture and antigen positivity has led to the concept of RADTs as an "infectiousness test." It has been proposed that viral culture may therefore be a more appropriate reference standard than PCR for asymptomatic testing. Nevertheless, this assumption is problematic as viral culture studies for SARS-CoV-

2 published to date lack standardization.[40] Preculture specimen handling (eg, storage at 4°C), as well as the cell line and culture protocol used, greatly impact the performance of culture.[41] Thus, although culture positivity indicates the presence of infectious virus, the absence of culture positivity itself does not definitively rule out the presence of infectious virus.

DIAGNOSTIC PERFORMANCE IN SYMPTOMATIC POPULATIONS

Performance characteristics of RADTs compared with PCR vary in published studies, likely due to differences in study design, PCR assay used, participant recruitment and demographics, and symptom duration. Although some RADT brands show solid performance characteristics, meta-analyses show a wide range of sensitivities among symptomatic patients (68.9% average sensitivity; 95% CI, 61.8%–75.1%).[42] Antigen testing specificity is generally high (99.6%; 95% CI, 99.0%–99.8%), though clusters of false-positive results have been described.[43] A summary of test performance among common brands is shown in **Table 1**.

Interpretation of studies regarding the performance of antigen testing among symptomatic patients can be challenging, even for assays considered to be among the most sensitive on the market. For example, among symptomatic participants at a community testing site in Wisconsin, the sensitivity of the Abbott BinaxNOW Ag Card (BinaxNOW) lateral flow immunoassay was 78.6% (95% CI, 73.4%–83.3%) compared with RT-PCR,[44] but was 95.4% (95% CI, 90.2%–98.3%) among symptomatic participants at a community testing site based in San Francisco[45] and 94.1% (95% CI, 71.1%–100%) at a similar site in the Netherlands.[46] Although some studies show high sensitivity for antigen testing in hospital settings, other studies have reported sensitivities as low as 66.4% (95% CI, 57.0%–74.9%).[47]

For assays that use digital readers, the Quidel SOFIA SARS Antigen Fluorescent Immunoassay (FIA) had 80.0% sensitivity (95% CI, 64.4%–90.9%) and 98.9% specificity (95% CI, 96.2%–99.9%) among symptomatic participants at 2 university campuses in Wisconsin, lower than what was reported in the FDA EUA.[48] A different study observed an 82% positive agreement with RT-PCR among symptomatic patients at an urgent care center.[28] The FIA also had comparable performance to the BD Veritor (Veritor) chromatographic digital immunoassay antigen test in specimens collected from drive-through and outpatient sites, despite apparent differences in sensitivity according to their respective EUA submission data.[49]

It is generally accepted that RADTs are unlikely to be positive beyond 7 days of symptoms, though this can differ somewhat by RADT brand (ie, 5 days vs 7 days). For example, the Innova assay remained positive for several days longer than the SureScreen F assay in one study.[31] Test performance may also be influenced by the number of symptoms present. For instance, the Veritor assay had 66.7% (95% CI, 30.0%–90.3%) positive agreement with PCR for patients with one symptom within 5 days of onset, compared with 88.0% (95% CI, 70.0%–95.8%) agreement among patients with at least 2 symptoms.[49]

RADT performance among pediatric patients has been variable between studies. Slightly lower concordance with RT-PCR was observed among children compared with adults (82% vs 85%, respectively).[50] Among symptomatic hospitalized kids, one study reported greater than 95% sensitivity for the PanBio assay,[51] but a much lower sensitivity of 45.4% (95% CI, 34.1%–57.2%) was observed in a different large multihospital study.[52] These divergent results may reflect differences in performance in adults versus children, regional differences in patient population, or differences in PCR methodology.

Table 1
Currently available FDA-cleared SARS-CoV-2 antigen tests[27]

Manufacturer	Test Name	Technology Used	Home-Use Option[a]	Indicated for Asymptomatic Testing	Separate Instrument Required	Performance Data for Detection of SARS-CoV-2
Abbott Diagnostics Scarborough, Inc	BinaxNOW COVID-19 Ag Card	Lateral flow immunoassay	No	No	No	PPA: 84.6% (76.8%–90.6%) NPA: 98.5% (96.6%–99.5%)
Abbott Diagnostics Scarborough, Inc	BinaxNOW COVID-19 Ag Card Home Test	Lateral flow immunoassay	Yes	No	Smartphone	PPA: 91.7% (73.0%–98.9%) NPA: 100.0% (87.7%–100.0%)
Abbott Diagnostics Scarborough, Inc	BinaxNOW COVID-19 Antigen Self Test	Lateral flow immunoassay	Yes	Yes	No	PPA: 91.7% (73.0%–98.9%) NPA: 100.0% (87.7%–100.0%)
Abbott Diagnostics Scarborough, Inc	BinaxNOW COVID-19 Ag Card 2 Home Test	Lateral flow immunoassay	Yes	Yes	Smartphone	PPA: 91.7% (73.0%–98.9%) NPA: 100.0% (87.7%–100.0%)
Abbott Diagnostics Scarborough, Inc	BinaxNOW COVID-19 Ag 2 Card	Lateral flow immunoassay	No	Yes	No	PPA: 84.6% (76.8%–90.6%) NPA: 98.5% (96.6%–99.5%)
Access Bio, Inc.	CareStart COVID-19 Antigen test	Lateral flow immunoassay	No	Yes	No	PPA: 93.75% (79.85%–98.27%) NPA: 99.32% (96.27%–99.88%)
ACON Laboratories, Inc.	Flowflex COVID-19 Antigen Home Test	Lateral flow immunoassay	Yes	Yes	No	PPA: 93% (81%–99%) NPA: 100% (97%–100%)
Becton, Dickinson and Company (BD)	BD Veritor System for Rapid Detection of SARS-CoV-2	Lateral flow immunoassay	No	Yes	No	PPA: 84% (67%–93%) NPA: 100% (98%–100%)
Becton, Dickinson and Company (BD)	BD Veritor System for Rapid Detection of SARS-CoV-2 & Flu A + B	Lateral flow immunoassay	No	No	No	PPA: 86.7% (75.8%–93.1%) NPA: 99.5% (97.4%–99.9%)

(continued on next page)

Table 1
(continued)

Manufacturer	Test Name	Technology Used	Home-Use Option[a]	Indicated for Asymptomatic Testing	Separate Instrument Required	Performance Data for Detection of SARS-CoV-2
Celltrion USA, Inc.	Celltrion DiaTrust COVID-19 Ag Rapid Test	Lateral flow immunoassay	No	Yes	No	PPA: 93.3% (78.7%–98.2%) NPA: 99.0% (94.7%–99.8%)
Celltrion USA, Inc.	Sampinute COVID-19 Antigen MIA	Magnetic force-assisted electrochemical sandwich immunoassay	No	No	Yes	PPA: 94.4% (80.0%–99.0%) NPA: 100.0% (88.0%–100.0%)
DiaSorin, Inc.	LIAISON SARS-CoV-2 Ag	Chemiluminescent immunoassay	No	No	No	PPA: 97.0% (84.7%–99.5%) NPA: 100% (96.6%–100%)
Ellume Limited	Ellume COVID-19 Home Test	Lateral flow immunoassay	Yes	Yes	No	PPA: 95% (82%–99%) NPA: 97% (93%–99%)
iHealth Labs, Inc.	iHealth COVID-19 Antigen Rapid Test Pro	Lateral flow immunoassay	No	No	No	PPA: 88.2% (73.4%–95.3%) NPA: 100% (88.6%–100%)
iHealth Labs, Inc.	iHealth COVID-19 Antigen Rapid Test	Lateral flow immunoassay	Yes	Yes	No	PPA: 94.3% (81.4%–98.4%) NPA: 98.1% (93.3%–99.5%)
InBios International, Inc.	SCoV-2 Ag Detect Rapid Test	Lateral flow immunoassay	No	Yes	No	PPA: 86.67% (73.82%–93.74%) NPA: 100% (98.53%–100.00%)
Luminostics, Inc.	Clip COVID Rapid Antigen Test	Lateral flow immunoluminescent assay	No	No	Yes	PPA: 96.96% (83.8%–99.9%) NPA: 100% (97.3%–100%)
LumiraDx UK Ltd.	LumiraDx SARS-CoV-2 Ag Test	Microfluidic immunofluorescence assay	No	No	Yes	PPA: 97.6% (91.6%–99.3%) NPA: 96.6% (92.7%–98.4%)
OraSure Technologies, Inc.	InteliiSwab COVID-19 Rapid Test Rx	Lateral flow immunoassay	Yes	No	No	PPA: 84% (71%–92%) NPA: 98% (93%–99%)

Manufacturer	Test	Method				Performance
OraSure Technologies, Inc.	IntelliSwab COVID-19 Rapid Test	Lateral flow immunoassay	Yes	Yes	No	PPA: 84% (71%–92%) NPA: 98% (93%–99%)
OraSure Technologies, Inc.	IntelliSwab COVID-19 Rapid Test Pro	Lateral flow immunoassay	No	Yes	No	PPA: 84% (71%–92%) NPA: 98% (93%–99%)
Ortho Clinical Diagnostics, Inc.	VITROS Immunodiagnostic Products SARS-CoV-2 Antigen Reagent Pack	Chemiluminescent immunoassay	No	No	Yes	PPA: 80.0% (56.6%–88.5%) NPA: 100.0% (95.2%–100.0%)
Princeton BioMeditech Corp	Status COVID-19/Flu	Lateral flow immunoassay	No	No	No	PPA: 93.9% (83.5%–97.9%) NPA: 100% (95.2%–100%)
Qorvo Biotechnologies, LLC	Omnia SARS-CoV-2 Antigen Test	Bulk acoustic wave biosensor	No	No	Yes	PPA: 89.47% (78.88%–95.09%) NPA: 100% (89.28%–100%)
Quanterix Corporation	Simoa SARS-CoV-2 N Protein Antigen Test	Paramagnetic microbead-based immunoassay	No	No	Yes	PPA: 97.7% (92.03%–99.72%) NPA: 100% (90.75%–100.0%)
Quidel Corporation	Sofia SARS Antigen FIA	Lateral flow immunofluorescence assay	No	Yes	Yes	PPA: 96.7% (83.3%–99.4%) NPA: 100% (97.9%–100.0%)
Quidel Corporation	Sofia 2 Flu + SARS Antigen FIA	Lateral flow immunofluorescence assay	No	No	Yes	PPA: 95.2% (84.2%–98.7%) NPA: 100.0% (96.9%–100.0%)
Quidel Corporation	QuickVue SARS Antigen Test	Lateral flow immunoassay	No	No	No	PPA: 96.6% (88.3%–99.0%) NPA: 99.3 (96.0%–99.9%)
Quidel Corporation	QuickVue At-Home COVID-19 Test	Lateral flow immunoassay	Yes	No	No	PPA: 84.8% (71.8%–92.4%) NPA: 99.1% (95.2%–99.8%)
Quidel Corporation	QuickVue At-Home OTC COVID-19 Test	Lateral flow immunoassay	Yes	Yes	No	PPA: 83.5% (74.9%–89.6%) NPA: 99.2% (97.2%–99.8%)
Salofa Oy	Sienna-Clarity COVID-19 Antigen Rapid Test Cassette	Lateral flow immunoassay	Yes	No	No	PPA: 87.5% (68.6%–93.0%) NPA: 98.9% (94.2%–99.9%)

[a] Over-the-counter or prescription required.

Symptomatic testing is arguably the most high-stakes application for RADTs. Antigen testing has limited utility in the diagnosis of symptomatic COVID-19 in hospital settings because patients who require hospitalization can present for evaluation after more than 1 week of symptoms. For this reason, they have been deemed to be unsuitable for rapid "rule-out" in an emergency department setting.[32,53] In nonhospital settings, however, the results of laboratory-based testing can take several days to return when demand is high, which makes it impractical for symptomatic people to isolate pending their test results. Thus, the primary benefit of a positive RADT result in symptomatic individuals in the community is the ability to facilitate immediate self-isolation when positive. However, low viral loads (and thus RADT-negativity) can occur during infection due to the natural course of illness, as well as due to suboptimal sample collection. Care must be taken to interpret tests in the context of symptoms and exposures, which both influence pretest probabilities. Finally, with the increasing prevalence of disease, it is important to remember that the negative predictive value of RADTs decreases.[3] Thus, the CDC currently recommends negative antigen results in the presence of symptoms should be confirmed with a molecular-based test.[54]

PERFORMANCE AS A TEST OF INFECTIOUSNESS IN ASYMPTOMATIC POPULATIONS

The ability of antigen testing to identify infectious asymptomatic or presymptomatic individuals, facilitating prompt self-isolation and breakage of transmission chains is an important application of this technology. RADT positivity drops steeply after infectious virus is no longer detected by cell culture, with a sensitivity of 23.8% at the end of 1 week of initial culture positivity compared with 85.7% for PCR in one study.[36] Antigen testing has therefore been suggested as a proxy for infectiousness; however, there is currently no infectiousness test for COVID-19 and the infectious dose of SARS-CoV-2 remains unknown. Detection of subgenomic (sg) RNA or minus-strand RNA indicates the presence of active viral replication and is generally interpreted as signifying that infectious virus may be present.[55] However, the relationship between sgRNA and culture positivity itself is somewhat controversial.[56] For better or worse, viral culture has become the de facto method for assessing infectiousness for COVID-19, with the limitations of viral culture having been discussed earlier.[57]

A major assumption has been that false-negative RADT results represent previously infected individuals with prolonged low-level detection by PCR. However, positivity by PCR generally can also precede RADT positivity by approximately 1 to 2 days,[31] and 75% of false-negative RADT results in one community study occurred among individuals who were presymptomatic.[50] In the same study, 11.8% of false-negative RADT specimens were culture positive with 53% being sgRNA positive. Thus, the proportion of false-negative RADT results that represent previous infection, rather presymptomatic infection (and thus potentially infectiousness), likely differs, depending on where in the epidemic curve a particular community is at that time because a greater proportion of people are early in the infection when cases are on the rise.[58]

For antigen testing to have utility as an "infectiousness test," one assumes that transmission is not generally readily observed among individuals with viral loads lower than what are reliably detected by RADTs. However, this does not necessarily appear to be the case. Firstly, significant overlap in Ct values occurs between spreaders and nonspreaders alike, including documented transmission by individuals with high Ct values.[59] Secondly, individuals with low viral loads, defined in one study as 1×10^6 copies/mL, had a secondary attack rate that was half that of individuals with high viral loads, but was still significant at 12%.[60] When the rate of local spread is high, the detection rate of RADTs for specimens with lower viral loads could potentially miss a sizable portion of presymptomatic and asymptomatic cases.[61]

Importantly, although the LoD of the BinaxNOW COVID-19 Antigen Card (Abbott, Scarborough, Maine) was shown to be approximately 4.0×10^4 to 8.1×10^4 copies per swab,[30] the LoD for several other RADT brands were shown to be much higher, at 2.1×10^6 to 2.9×10^7 per swab.[62] As such, transmission can and does occur among individuals with viral loads that could reasonably be expected to test negative by RADTs. Critically, transmission dynamics are influenced by several factors beyond solely viral load; these include the contact pattern (eg, duration of exposure, activity), host factors (eg, age), and the environment (eg, ventilation).[63] Thus, a negative RADT result in an asymptomatic individual should not be thought of as a definitive statement on noninfectiousness, but rather, indicating likely noninfectiousness at the time of sampling.

Initial modeling data suggested that more frequent serial testing can mitigate concerns over RADT sensitivity[64,65] because the sensitivity of antigen testing before the first day of detectable shedding of infectious virus was 37.5% compared with 65% for RT-PCR. For this reason, FDA EUAs for asymptomatic testing specify that serial testing should be performed. Recently, 2 studies using real-world data have confirmed the results of initial modeling studies. In a large study among college students, weekly nasal PCR testing had a sensitivity of 98.7% for COVID-19 screening detection, with comparable sensitivities for RADTs (>98%) performed every third day, dropping to 79.7% when performed only weekly.[66] During an intercollegiate program of daily RADT and weekly paired PCR/antigen testing (81,175 and 23,462 tests, respectively), daily antigen testing had similar sensitivities to twice-to-thrice weekly PCR testing.[67]

At face value, it could be argued asymptomatic testing has few downsides because any case detected is one that would otherwise have not been detected. From this perspective, the tests are viewed as a public health intervention rather than as a diagnostic, which was their intended design.[68,69] However, false-negative test results have clinical consequences for the individual and can also influence the behavior of the test recipient in a fashion that promotes spread of the virus to others. A negative test result (whether PCR or antigen) is not a replacement for other public health measures and the same considerations that influence test performance in symptomatic individuals (eg, specimen quality, timing of testing) are similarly a consideration in this setting.

An additional concern is that even a test with excellent specificity will have a poor positive predictive value (PPV) during periods of low infection prevalence.[70,71] For example, PPV is predicted to be only 28.8% for a test with 98% specificity when disease prevalence is 1%.[72] This was also shown in a real-world study where a 66.7% false-positivity rate was noted for RADTs.[48] A different study performed in August 2020 reported that 23 of 39 (60%) of samples positive by RADT were negative by RT-PCR across several skilled nursing facilities.[73] The reasons for this cluster of false positives were never fully determined but could represent issues with poor quality test manufacturing. Concerns over test specificity can be mitigated by requiring positive results in asymptomatic people to be confirmed by secondary testing, which is recommended by the current CDC interim guidelines.[54] However, such confirmation may not necessarily be required when community infection rates are high. It is therefore important to continually reevaluate the prevalence of infection in a region where antigen testing will be implemented. Unfortunately, as in-home RADT becomes more available in the United States, a system for linkage to confirmatory PCR testing and to public health surveillance systems continues to be lacking, which leads to underestimates of disease prevalence.

ASYMPTOMATIC ANTIGEN TESTING IN PRACTICE

Several studies modeled the potential impact of widespread antigen testing to screen asymptomatic populations, with some even factoring in behaviors such as unwillingness to test or isolate.[64,65,74] One study predicted that with a test sensitivity of 80%, weekly testing would prevent almost 3 million cases and over 16,000 deaths in the United States.[74] There are 5 main areas where asymptomatic antigen testing has been applied in practice and we will review each of these applications here.

Antigen Testing as a Circuit Breaker

Mass population testing has been implemented by some governments in an attempt to halt exponential increases in case numbers. RADT testing with swabs collected under supervision from military personnel was used in a large-scale community testing initiative over 6 months in the city of Liverpool. This intervention led to an estimated 18% increase (95% CI, 7%–29%) in case detection, a 21% reduction (95% CI, 12%–27%) in cases during the first 6 weeks compared with control areas, but had no significant impact on the number of hospital admissions.[75] Notably, in interviews with participants who chose not to test, the biggest barriers to participation were fear of income loss, skepticism over the need to test, as well as crowded and inconvenient waiting lines.[75]

Arguably, it is Slovakia's experience that has driven the narrative about the power of mass antigen testing to halt case surges. The results from Slovakia are indeed striking: after one round of mass antigen testing, the prevalence of SARS-CoV-2 decreased by 58% (95 CI, 57%–58%). In districts that had a positivity rate ≥ 0.7%, a second round of testing was performed, after which a 0.3 decrease in the reproductive number (ie, R0) occurred 2 weeks later.[76] Mass antigen testing revealed 5594 cases compared with only 782 cases that would have otherwise been identified by routine clinical testing. Disease prevalence decreased from 3.97% to 1% 1 week later with modeling data suggesting that 46,137 infections were prevented as a result of the program.[77]

Importantly, mass antigen testing was not the sole public health intervention used by the Slovakian government; noncompliance in the testing program required a 10-day home quarantine, with random police inspections and a fine equivalent to $1.5\times$ the national monthly wage issued for those caught breaking quarantine. Other measures implemented included limiting gatherings of more than 50 people and closure of restaurants and schools.[78] Though it was concluded that frequent mass testing would be necessary to sustain the decrease in cases, nevertheless, the Slovakian experience shows the potential of mass testing when combined with other measures. In practice, such measures would likely be considered unpalatable to a significant proportion of the US populace.

Daily Testing to Enable Close Contact

Daily antigen testing with the SOFIA assay (Quidel, San Diego, California), in addition to weekly PCR testing, was implemented by universities in the United States to facilitate the continuation of intercollegiate sports programs.[67] In all, 172 athletes had SARS-CoV-2 detected, with 52% identified as positive on days between weekly PCR tests. In all, 234 days of potential infectiousness were avoided as a result of the daily antigen testing program. There were also 98 false-positive RADT results, but negative impact was minimized by ready access to PCR results with rapid turnaround time.

The authors observed that antigen positivity lagged about 1 day behind PCR detection. Even with nurse-supervised specimen collection, daily antigen testing failed to prevent outbreaks on 2 occasions involving a total of 32 individuals.[79] PCR results were available for the initial false-negative RADT result in 1 of the 2 index cases: despite a low Ct value of 15.9, the patient tested negative by RADT but subsequently developed symptoms later the same day. Mass PCR testing was performed 7 times during these outbreaks, leading to the identification of 21 new cases, 86% of whom were antigen negative. The most likely reason for the false-negative antigen test results in contact tracing networks is due to individuals being too early in their infection curve to be detectable by RADTs. In support of this, transmission was only interrupted when serial PCR was performed during the outbreak to identify additional cases. The study's authors concluded that *"serial antigen testing may have limited sensitivity for detecting early asymptomatic infections,"*[79] suggesting a two-tier strategy of antigen tests backed by intensive PCR sampling as the optimal approach for surveillance and containment.

To Attend Events or to Travel

The utility of day-of-testing to attend live, indoor concerts was investigated in 2 studies conducted in Catalonia, Spain. Attendees were tested using the Panbio assay (Abbott, Scarborough, Maine) before entry at a live music concert. Follow-up studies 8 days later showed no difference in COVID-19 incidence between the control and intervention groups.[80] Importantly, concertgoers were required to wear N95 face masks, the venue was well-ventilated, and there were restrictions on direction of movement and crowding in smaller spaces. In a follow-up study by the same group looking at a 5000-person event using the same combination of additional public health measures, 6 RADT positive and likely infectious individuals, along with 2 of their close contacts, were prevented from attending the concert.[81] Only 6 cases were diagnosed within 2 weeks of the event, 3 of whom were identified as being close contacts of COVID-19 case who did not attend the concert. Although it is not possible to discern the specific impact of antigen testing per se, both studies showed that mass day-of-event RADT testing, when combined with masking and adequate ventilation, facilitates normalization of activity and mass gatherings.

Day-of-testing was also used to screen passengers at 2 major US airports before and immediately after their flights.[82] Antigen testing detected 4 individuals (0.04%), who tested positive by both antigen testing and confirmatory RT-PCR.[82] Concerningly, as infection prevalence was estimated to be low at 1.1% at the time, there were 12 false-positive rapid antigen tests results out of 9849 total tested that did not confirm by RT-PCR.[82] This testing occurred in addition to other interventions already in place, for example, masking, vaccination, and distancing.

Postexposure Testing in Schools

RADTs have been tool to limit SARS-CoV-2 transmission in schools. In a randomized study involving secondary schools and colleges, students and staff with known exposure to an infected contact were either required to self-isolate for 10 days (control group) or given the option to continue attending school provided with daily RADT testing (intervention group).[83] Overall positivity postexposure was low at ~2% in both groups, and the impact of RADT alone is difficult to assess as other safety precautions were in place, for example, masking. School absences were also not significantly reduced in the intervention group.[83]

Performance of At-Home Testing

Though some governments have provided at-home testing to their residents free-of-charge (eg, the United Kingdom and the United States), the overwhelming majority of studies to date on antigen testing involve performance by trained staff.[45,84] The performance of at-home RADTs is relatively understudied by comparison. Though studies show only minor differences in performance between health care worker (HCW)-collected and HCW-supervised specimen collection,[85] the performance of at-home, unsupervised specimen collection may differ. In a study looking at the performance of SARS-CoV-2 RT-PCR, home-collected specimens had a sensitivity of 80% compared with clinician-collected swabs[86]; such differences would also be expected to apply to RADTs. Similarly, testing performed by laboratory scientists was 78.8% sensitive compared with fully trained research HCWs (70%), with both groups exceeding the sensitivity of self-trained members of the public (57.5%).[28] Rates of positivity were similar between the different collectors for specimens with low Ct values, but differences became more pronounced for specimens with Ct values in the 25–28 range.[28] Finally, one infrequently discussed element with regards to at-home testing is the potential for test transportation/shipping conditions to deleteriously impact test performance. False-negative results were noted when test kits stored at high temperatures, with false-positive results observed with lower temperatures.[87]

CONCLUSIONS AND FUTURE CONSIDERATIONS
Variants

Antigen testing appears to thus far be unaffected by the emergence of SARS-CoV-2 variants at least with respect to the performance of the BinaxNOW (Abbott) assay, showing equivalent performance for major variants including the Delta variant (B.1.617)[88] and Omicron variant (B.1.429).[89,90] The performance of other RADT brands is unknown as of the time of writing. Importantly, Bourassa and colleagues observed that SARS-CoV-2 specimens with a D399N nucleocapsid mutation were not detected by the SOFIA assay but were detected by the BinaxNOW test.[91] Thus, continued investigation on the part of the RADT manufacturers and independent researchers will be necessary to ensure that a given RADT brand continues to perform equivalently as new variants continue to emerge.

Impact of Variants on Kinetics of Antigen Positivity

An average of 4.3 days transpires between the beginning of viral shedding and peak viral load with the alpha variant (B1.1.7).[92] In contrast, the time from exposure to detection was reduced to 3 days with the Delta variant compared with 6 days for the wild-type strain.[93] Whether the shortened time it takes for variants to reach peak viral loads warrants a reconsideration of the frequency of serial RADT testing is currently unknown.

Vaccine Breakthrough Cases

Though vaccination reduces the incidence of both asymptomatic and asymptomatic infection even against variants,[94] breakthrough cases with the Delta variant in vaccinated patients had initial Ct values that were indistinguishable from those occurring in unvaccinated individuals.[95] The duration of antigen positivity in vaccinated individuals has not been well defined; however, in a study with HCWs, culturable virus was less likely to be recovered from vaccinated HCWs with breakthrough Delta variant infection compared with unvaccinated infected HCWs at 68.6% versus 84.9%, respectively.[96] Whether antigen positivity mirrors culture positivity among vaccinated individuals with breakthrough infection remains to be determined.

Public Health Reporting

There is generally a lack of structured or automated result reporting to public health authorities for surveillance for many RADTs. In a Kaiser Health News survey, nearly half of US states indicated antigen test results are underreported.[97] This can lead to missed opportunities for contact tracing and inaccuracies in tracking positivity rates and potential outbreaks. Furthermore, laboratories are unable to easily follow-up on positive samples for sequencing. This may hamper efforts to detect and track potential variants of concern as they emerge.[98]

Parting Thoughts

The promise of antigen testing is fundamentally associated with its ability to democratize testing, enabling rapid detection of both asymptomatic and symptomatic infection alike and breakage of transmission chains. Nevertheless, the narrative of using RADTs to know one's "infectious status" does not reflect the nuance of testing, that is, that such a status is not static and that transmission among individuals with low viral loads occurs. It is when RADT positivity and contagiousness match that they can have the greatest impact; however, it is often the case that there is a mismatch between the two .

Although it has been proposed that RADTs be considered "public health tests" that are separate from their role as clinical diagnostics, they will invariably be used by symptomatic individuals for personal decision making because results have implications on the health of the test recipient. What has been fundamentally absent in the United States is concerted government-led education around how RADTs should be used and how results should be interpreted along with linkage to confirmatory and timely PCR testing. Unlocking the true power of this technology requires sufficient and cheap/free test supply and sufficient understanding among the general public of its limitations. This may be changing with the free distribution by the US government of RADTs to individuals who request them using an online portal.[99] As we have highlighted in this review, a multitude of data show that antigen testing works best when used as one element of a coordinated strategy involving vaccination and nonpharmacologic interventions, and not as the sole intervention. Indeed, there are no data published on the impact of frequent RADT surveillance in the absence of other public health measures.

Ultimately, although the promise of antigen testing for SARS-CoV-2 comes from their massive scale, it has been frequently conveyed as if its power comes from individual decision-making. If the true potential of antigen testing is to be harnessed, society would do well to remember the original motto of the United States proposed by the founding fathers: "*E pluribus unum,*" or "*out of many, one.*" There is no singular solution to ending this pandemic, but certainly, the true power of antigen technology will come from its combination with other public health measures.

REFERENCES

1. Ranney ML, Griffeth V, Jha AK. Critical supply shortages - the need for ventilators and personal protective equipment during the Covid-19 Pandemic. N Engl J Med 2020;382(18):e41.

2. Hanson Kimberly E, Caliendo Angela M, Arias Cesar A, et al. Infectious Diseases Society of America Guidelines on the Diagnosis of COVID-19. Available at: https://www.idsociety.org/practice-guideline/covid-19-guideline-diagnostics/. Accessed October 2, 2021.

3. Scaling up COVID-19 rapid antigen tests: promises and challenges - the Lancet Infectious Diseases. Available at: https://www.thelancet.com/journals/laninf/article/PIIS1473-3099(21)00048-7/fulltext. Accessed October 2, 2021.

4. Cevik M, Tate M, Lloyd O, et al. SARS-CoV-2, SARS-CoV, and MERS-CoV viral load dynamics, duration of viral shedding, and infectiousness: a systematic review and meta-analysis. Lancet Microbe 2021;2(1):e13–22.

5. Prince-Guerra JL, Almendares O, Nolen LD, et al. Evaluation of Abbott Binax-NOW rapid antigen test for SARS-CoV-2 infection at two community-based testing sites — Pima County, Arizona, November 3–17, 2020. MMWR Morb Mortal Wkly Rep 2021;70(3):100–5.

6. Pekosz A, Parvu V, Li M, et al. Antigen-based testing but not real-time polymerase chain reaction correlates with severe acute respiratory syndrome Coronavirus 2 viral culture. Clin Infect Dis 2021. https://doi.org/10.1093/cid/ciaa1706. ciaa1706.

7. Ginocchio CC, Zhang F, Manji R, et al. Evaluation of multiple test methods for the detection of the novel 2009 influenza A (H1N1) during the New York City outbreak. J Clin Virol 2009;45(3):191–5.

8. Accuracy of rapid influenza diagnostic tests: a meta-analysis: Ann Intern Med: Vol 156, No 7. Available at: https://www.acpjournals.org/doi/full/10.7326/0003-4819-156-7-201204030-00403?rfr_dat=cr_pub++0pubmed&url_ver=Z39.88-2003&rfr_id=ori%3Arid%3Acrossref.org. Accessed October 2, 2021.

9. Merckx J, Wali R, Schiller I, et al. Diagnostic accuracy of novel and traditional rapid tests for influenza infection compared with reverse transcriptase polymerase chain reaction. Ann Intern Med 2017;167(6):394–409.

10. Pinsky BA, Hayden RT. Cost-effective respiratory virus testing. J Clin Microbiol 2019;57(9):e00373-19.

11. Rapid influenza diagnostic tests | CDC. 2019. Available at: https://www.cdc.gov/flu/professionals/diagnosis/clinician_guidance_ridt.htm. Accessed October 2, 2021.

12. Occurrence and transmission potential of asymptomatic and presymptomatic SARS-CoV-2 infections: a living systematic review and meta-analysis. Available at: https://www.ncbi.nlm.nih.gov/pmc/articles/PMC7508369/. Accessed October 2, 2021.

13. Lau LLH, Cowling BJ, Fang VJ, et al. Viral shedding and clinical illness in naturally acquired influenza virus infections. J Infect Dis 2010;201(10):1509–16.

14. Ip DKM, Lau LLH, Leung NHL, et al. Viral shedding and transmission potential of asymptomatic and paucisymptomatic influenza virus infections in the community. Clin Infect Dis 2017;64(6):736–42.

15. Suess T, Remschmidt C, Schink SB, et al. Comparison of shedding characteristics of seasonal influenza virus (Sub)Types and influenza A(H1N1)pdm09; Germany, 2007–2011. PLoS One 2012;7(12):e51653.

16. AF, BaligaChris, AklPascale, et al. Pre-procedural Covid-19 screening of asymptomatic patients: a model for protecting patients, community and staff during expansion of surgical care. NEJM catalyst innovations in care delivery. 2020. Available at: https://catalyst.nejm.org/doi/full/10.1056/cat.20.0261. Accessed October 2, 2021.

17. Krüger S, Leskien M, Schuller P, et al. Performance and feasibility of universal PCR admission screening for SARS-CoV-2 in a German tertiary care hospital. J Med Virol 2021;93(5):2890–8.

18. He X, Lau EHY, Wu P, et al. Temporal dynamics in viral shedding and transmissibility of COVID-19. Nat Med 2020;26(5):672–5.

19. Khoshchehreh M, Wald-Dickler N, Holtom P, et al. A needle in the haystack? Assessing the significance of envelope (E) gene-negative, nucleocapsid (N2) gene-positive SARS-CoV-2 detection by the Cepheid Xpert Xpress SARS-COV-2 assay. J Clin Virol 2020;133:104683.

20. Chandler CM, Bourassa L, Mathias PC, et al. Estimating the false-positive rate of highly automated SARS-CoV-2 nucleic acid amplification testing. J Clin Microbiol 2021;59(8):e0108021.

21. Lin L, Carlquist J, Sinclair W, et al. Experience with false-positive test results on the TaqPath real-time reverse transcription-polymerase chain reaction Coronavirus Disease 2019 (COVID-19) testing platform. Arch Pathol Lab Med 2021; 145(3):259–61.

22. Health C for D and R. Potential for false positive results with Abbott Molecular Inc. Alinity m SARS-CoV-2 AMP and Alinity m Resp-4-Plex AMP kits - Letter to clinical laboratory staff and health care Providers. FDA. 2021. Available at: https://www.fda.gov/medical-devices/letters-health-care-providers/potential-false-positive-results-abbott-molecular-inc-alinity-m-sars-cov-2-amp-and-alinity-m-resp-4. Accessed October 2, 2021.

23. Stokes W, Berenger BM, Portnoy D, et al. Clinical performance of the Abbott Panbio with nasopharyngeal, throat, and saliva swabs among symptomatic individuals with COVID-19. Eur J Clin Microbiol Infect Dis 2021;1–6. https://doi.org/10.1007/s10096-021-04202-9.

24. Uwamino Y, Nagata M, Aoki W, et al. Accuracy of rapid antigen detection test for nasopharyngeal swab specimens and saliva samples in comparison with RT-PCR and viral culture for SARS-CoV-2 detection. J Infect Chemother 2021;27(7): 1058–62.

25. Manabe YC, Reuland C, Yu T, et al. Self-collected oral fluid saliva is insensitive compared with nasal-oropharyngeal swabs in the detection of severe acute respiratory syndrome Coronavirus 2 in outpatients. Open Forum Infect Dis 2021;8(2): ofaa648.

26. Yokota I, Shane PY, Okada K, et al. A novel strategy for SARS-CoV-2 mass screening with quantitative antigen testing of saliva: a diagnostic accuracy study. Lancet Microbe 2021;2(8):e397–404.

27. Health C for D and R. In vitro diagnostics EUAs - antigen diagnostic tests for SARS-CoV-2. FDA. 2021. Available at: https://www.fda.gov/medical-devices/coronavirus-disease-2019-covid-19-emergency-use-authorizations-medical-devices/in-vitro-diagnostics-euas-antigen-diagnostic-tests-sars-cov-2. Accessed October 2, 2021.

28. Peto T, Affron D, Afrough B, et al. COVID-19: rapid antigen detection for SARS-CoV-2 by lateral flow assay: a national systematic evaluation of sensitivity and specificity for mass-testing. EClinicalMedicine 2021;36. https://doi.org/10.1016/j.eclinm.2021.100924.

29. Protocol for evaluation of rapid diagnostic assays for specific SARS-CoV-2 antigens (lateral flow devices). GOV.UK. Available at: https://www.gov.uk/government/publications/assessment-and-procurement-of-coronavirus-covid-19-tests/protocol-for-evaluation-of-rapid-diagnostic-assays-for-specific-sars-cov-2-antigens-lateral-flow-devices. Accessed October 2, 2021.

30. Perchetti GA, Huang ML, Mills MG, et al. Analytical sensitivity of the Abbott Binax-NOW COVID-19 Ag card. J Clin Microbiol 2021;59(3):e02880-20.

31. Pickering S, Batra R, Merrick B, et al. Comparative performance of SARS-CoV-2 lateral flow antigen tests and association with detection of infectious virus in clinical specimens: a single-centre laboratory evaluation study. Lancet Microbe 2021;2(9):e461–71.

32. Holzner C, Pabst D, Anastasiou OE, et al. SARS-CoV-2 rapid antigen test: fast-safe or dangerous? An analysis in the emergency department of an university hospital. J Med Virol 2021. https://doi.org/10.1002/jmv.27033.

33. Rhoads DD, Pinsky BA. The truth about SARS-CoV-2 cycle threshold values is rarely pure and never simple. Clin Chem 2021;hvab146. https://doi.org/10.1093/clinchem/hvab146.

34. Richard-Greenblatt M, Ziegler MJ, Bromberg V, et al. Quantifying the impact of nasopharyngeal specimen quality on severe acute respiratory syndrome coronavirus 2 test performance. Open Forum Infect Dis 2021;8(6). https://doi.org/10.1093/ofid/ofab235.

35. Singanayagam A, Patel M, Charlett A, et al. Duration of infectiousness and correlation with RT-PCR cycle threshold values in cases of COVID-19, England, January to May 2020. Euro Surveill 2020;25(32):2001483.

36. Walsh KA, Spillane S, Comber L, et al. The duration of infectiousness of individuals infected with SARS-CoV-2. J Infect 2020;0(0). https://doi.org/10.1016/j.jinf.2020.10.009.

37. Folgueira MD, Luczkowiak J, Lasala F, et al. Prolonged SARS-CoV-2 cell culture replication in respiratory samples from patients with severe COVID-19. Clin Microbiol Infect 2021;27(6):886–91.

38. Aydillo T, Gonzalez-Reiche AS, Aslam S, et al. Shedding of viable SARS-CoV-2 after immunosuppressive therapy for cancer. N Engl J Med 2020. https://doi.org/10.1056/NEJMc2031670. NEJMc2031670.

39. Truong TT, Ryutov A, Pandey U, et al. Increased viral variants in children and young adults with impaired humoral immunity and persistent SARS-CoV-2 infection: a consecutive case series. EBioMedicine 2021;67:103355.

40. Jefferson T, Spencer EA, Brassey J, et al. Viral cultures for COVID-19 infectious potential assessment - a systematic review. Clin Infect Dis 2020;ciaa1764. https://doi.org/10.1093/cid/ciaa1764.

41. Wurtz N, Penant G, Jardot P, et al. Culture of SARS-CoV-2 in a panel of laboratory cell lines, permissivity, and differences in growth profile. Eur J Clin Microbiol Infect Dis 2021;40(3):477–84.

42. Dinnes J, Deeks JJ, Berhane S, et al. Rapid, point-of-care antigen and molecular-based tests for diagnosis of SARS-CoV-2 infection. Cochrane Database Syst Rev 2021;(3). https://doi.org/10.1002/14651858.CD013705.pub2.

43. A tale of two tests: vermont town left puzzled by positive, then negative, COVID-19 results - the Boston Globe. Available at: https://www.bostonglobe.com/2020/07/22/nation/tale-two-tests-vermont-city-left-puzzled-by-positive-then-negative-covid-19-results/. Accessed October 2, 2021.

44. Shah MM, Salvatore PP, Ford L, et al. Performance of repeat BinaxNOW SARS-CoV-2 antigen testing in a community setting, Wisconsin, november-december 2020. Clin Infect Dis 2021;ciab309. https://doi.org/10.1093/cid/ciab309.

45. Pilarowski G, Marquez C, Rubio L, et al. Field performance and public health response using the BinaxNOW TM Rapid SARS-CoV-2 antigen detection assay during community-based testing. Clin Infect Dis 2020;ciaa1890. https://doi.org/10.1093/cid/ciaa1890.

46. Van der Moeren N, Zwart VF, Lodder EB, et al. Evaluation of the test accuracy of a SARS-CoV-2 rapid antigen test in symptomatic community dwelling individuals in The Netherlands. PLoS One 2021;16(5):e0250886.

47. Kilic A, Hiestand B, Palavecino E. Evaluation of performance of the BD Veritor SARS-CoV-2 chromatographic immunoassay test in patients with symptoms of COVID-19. J Clin Microbiol 2021;59(5):e00260-21.

48. Pray IW, Ford L, Cole D, et al. Performance of an antigen-based test for asymptomatic and symptomatic SARS-CoV-2 testing at two university campuses -

Wisconsin, september-october 2020. MMWR Morb Mortal Wkly Rep 2021; 69(5152):1642–7.

49. Young S, Taylor SN, Cammarata CL, et al. Clinical evaluation of BD Veritor SARS-CoV-2 point-of-care test performance compared to PCR-based testing and versus the sofia 2 SARS antigen point-of-care test. J Clin Microbiol 2020;59(1): e02338-20.

50. Ford L, Whaley MJ, Shah MM, et al. Antigen test performance among children and adults at a SARS-CoV-2 community testing site. J Pediatr Infect Dis Soc 2021. https://doi.org/10.1093/jpids/piab081. piab081.

51. Eleftheriou I, Dasoula F, Dimopoulou D, et al. Real-life evaluation of a COVID-19 rapid antigen detection test in hospitalized children. J Med Virol 2021;93(10): 6040–4.

52. Villaverde S, Domínguez-Rodríguez S, Sabrido G, et al. Diagnostic accuracy of the panbio severe acute respiratory syndrome coronavirus 2 antigen rapid test compared with reverse-transcriptase polymerase chain reaction testing of naso-pharyngeal samples in the pediatric population. J Pediatr 2021;232:287–9.e4.

53. Osterman A, Baldauf HM, Eletreby M, et al. Evaluation of two rapid antigen tests to detect SARS-CoV-2 in a hospital setting. Med Microbiol Immunol 2021;210(1): 65–72.

54. CDC. Interim Guidelines for Collecting, Handling, and Testing Clinical Specimens for COVID-19. Centers for Disease Control and Prevention. 2020. Available at: https://www.cdc.gov/coronavirus/2019-ncov/lab/guidelines-clinical-specimens.html. Accessed February 21, 2021.

55. Hogan CA, Huang C, Sahoo MK, et al. Strand-specific reverse transcription PCR for detection of replicating SARS-CoV-2. Emerg Infect Dis 2021. https://doi.org/10.3201/eid2702.204168.

56. Binnicker MJ. Can testing predict SARS-CoV-2 infectivity? The potential for certain methods to be a surrogate for replication-competent virus. J Clin Microbiol 2021. https://doi.org/10.1128/JCM.00469-21. JCM0046921.

57. Brümmer LE, Katzenschlager S, Gaeddert M, et al. Accuracy of novel antigen rapid diagnostics for SARS-CoV-2: a living systematic review and meta-analysis. PLOS Med 2021;18(8):e1003735.

58. Hay JA, Kennedy-Shaffer L, Kanjilal S, et al. Estimating epidemiologic dynamics from cross-sectional viral load distributions. Science 2021;373(6552). https://doi.org/10.1126/science.abh0635.

59. Tian D, Lin Z, Kriner EM, et al. Ct values do not predict severe acute respiratory syndrome Coronavirus 2 (SARS-CoV-2) transmissibility in college students. J Mol Diagn 2021;23(9):1078–84.

60. Marks M, Millat-Martinez P, Ouchi D, et al. Transmission of COVID-19 in 282 clusters in Catalonia, Spain: a cohort study. Lancet Infect Dis 2021;21(5):629–36.

61. Wan Z, Zhao Y, Lu R, et al. Rapid antigen detection alone may not be sufficient for early diagnosis and/or mass screening of COVID-19. J Med Virol 2021. https://doi.org/10.1002/jmv.27236.

62. Corman VM, Haage VC, Bleicker T, et al. Comparison of seven commercial SARS-CoV-2 rapid point-of-care antigen tests: a single-centre laboratory evaluation study. Lancet Microbe 2021;2(7):e311–9.

63. Cevik M, Marcus JL, Buckee C, et al. Severe acute respiratory syndrome Coronavirus 2 (SARS-CoV-2) transmission dynamics should inform policy. Clin Infect Dis 2021;73(Suppl 2):S170–6.

64. Larremore DB, Wilder B, Lester E, et al. Test sensitivity is secondary to frequency and turnaround time for COVID-19 screening. Sci Adv 2021;7(1):eabd5393.

65. See I, Paul P, Slayton RB, et al. Modeling effectiveness of testing strategies to prevent Coronavirus disease 2019 (COVID-19) in nursing homes—United States, 2020. Clin Infect Dis 2021;73(3):e792–8.

66. Smith RL, Gibson LL, Martinez PP, et al. Longitudinal assessment of diagnostic test performance over the course of acute SARS-CoV-2 Infection. J Infect Dis 2021;224(6):976–82.

67. Harmon K, de St Maurice AM, Brady AC, et al. Surveillance testing for SARS-COV-2 infection in an asymptomatic athlete population: a prospective cohort study with 123 362 tests and 23 463 paired RT-PCR/antigen samples. BMJ Open Sport Exerc Med 2021;7(2):e001137.

68. Ricks S, Kendall EA, Dowdy DW, et al. Quantifying the potential value of antigen-detection rapid diagnostic tests for COVID-19: a modelling analysis. BMC Med 2021;19(1):75.

69. Schwartz KL, McGeer AJ, Bogoch II. Rapid antigen screening of asymptomatic people as a public health tool to combat COVID-19. CMAJ 2021;193(13): E449–52.

70. García-Fiñana M, Buchan IE. Rapid antigen testing in COVID-19 responses. Science 2021;372(6542):571–2.

71. Health C for D and R. Potential for false positive results with antigen tests for rapid detection of SARS-CoV-2 - Letter to clinical laboratory staff and health care Providers. FDA. 2020. Available at: https://www.fda.gov/medical-devices/letters-health-care-providers/potential-false-positive-results-antigen-tests-rapid-detection-sars-cov-2-letter-clinical-laboratory. Accessed October 2, 2021.

72. Pettengill MA, McAdam AJ. Can we test our way out of the COVID-19 Pandemic? J Clin Microbiol 2020;58(11):e02225-20.

73. Azzam Ihsan, Pandori Mark, Sherych Lisa. Discontinue the use of antigen testing in skilled nursing facilities until further notice. 2020. Available at: https://dpbh.nv.gov/uploadedFiles/dpbhnvgov/content/Resources/Directive%20to%20Discontinue%20Use%20of%20Antigen%20POC_10.02.2020_ADA_Compliant.pdf. Accessed February 14, 2022.

74. Paltiel AD, Zheng A, Sax PE. Clinical and economic effects of widespread rapid testing to decrease SARS-CoV-2 Transmission. Ann Intern Med 2021;174(6): 803–10.

75. University of Liverpool. Liverpool Covid-SMART community testing Pilot evaluation Report.;. 2021. Available at: https://www.liverpool.ac.uk/coronavirus/research-and-analysis/covid-smart-pilot/. Accessed October 4, 2021.

76. Kahanec M, Lafférs L, Schmidpeter B. The impact of repeated mass antigen testing for COVID-19 on the prevalence of the disease. J Popul Econ 2021;1–36. https://doi.org/10.1007/s00148-021-00856-z.

77. Frnda J, Durica M. On Pilot massive COVID-19 testing by antigen tests in Europe. Case study: Slovakia. Infect Dis Rep 2021;13(1):45–57.

78. Pavelka M, Van-Zandvoort K, Abbott S, et al. The impact of population-wide rapid antigen testing on SARS-CoV-2 prevalence in Slovakia. Science 2021;372(6542): 635–41.

79. Moreno GK, Braun KM, Pray IW, et al. Severe Acute Respiratory Syndrome Coronavirus 2 transmission in intercollegiate athletics not fully mitigated with daily antigen testing. Clin Infect Dis 2021;73(Suppl 1):S45–53.

80. Revollo B, Blanco I, Soler P, et al. Same-day SARS-CoV-2 antigen test screening in an indoor mass-gathering live music event: a randomised controlled trial. Lancet Infect Dis 2021;21(10):1365–72.

81. Llibre JM, Videla S, Clotet B, et al. Screening for SARS-CoV-2 antigen before a live indoor music concert: an observational study. Ann Intern Med 2021. https://doi.org/10.7326/M21-2278.

82. Tande AJ, Binnicker MJ, Ting HH, et al. SARS-CoV-2 testing prior to International Airline Travel, december 2020-may 2021. Mayo Clin Proc 2021. https://doi.org/10.1016/j.mayocp.2021.08.019.

83. Young BC, Eyre DW, Kendrick S, et al. Daily testing for contacts of individuals with SARS-CoV-2 infection and attendance and SARS-CoV-2 transmission in English secondary schools and colleges: an open-label, cluster-randomised trial. Lancet 2021;398(10307):1217–29.

84. Pollock NR, Jacobs JR, Tran K, et al. Performance and implementation evaluation of the Abbott BinaxNOW rapid antigen test in a high-throughput drive-through community testing site in Massachusetts. J Clin Microbiol 2021;59(5):e00083-21.

85. Klein JAF, Krüger LJ, Tobian F, et al. Head-to-head performance comparison of self-collected nasal versus professional-collected nasopharyngeal swab for a WHO-listed SARS-CoV-2 antigen-detecting rapid diagnostic test. Med Microbiol Immunol 2021;210(4):181–6.

86. McCulloch DJ, Kim AE, Wilcox NC, et al. Comparison of unsupervised home self-collected midnasal swabs with clinician-collected nasopharyngeal swabs for detection of SARS-CoV-2 Infection. JAMA Netw Open 2020;3(7):e2016382.

87. Haage V, Ferreira de Oliveira-Filho E, Moreira-Soto A, et al. Impaired performance of SARS-CoV-2 antigen-detecting rapid diagnostic tests at elevated and low temperatures. J Clin Virol 2021;138:104796.

88. Frediani JK, Levy JM, Rao A, et al. Multidisciplinary assessment of the Abbott BinaxNOW SARS-CoV-2 point-of-care antigen test in the context of emerging viral variants and self-administration. Sci Rep 2021;11(1):14604.

89. Kanjilal S, Chalise S, Shah AS, et al. Analytic Sensitivity of the Abbott BinaxNOWTM Lateral Flow Immunochromatographic Assay for the SARS-CoV-2 Omicron Variant.; 2022. doi:10.1101/2022.01.10.22269033

90. Deerain J, Druce J, Tran T, et al. Assessment of the analytical sensitivity of ten lateral flow devices against the SARS-CoV-2 omicron variant. J Clin Microbiol 2021;60(2). e02479–21.

91. Bourassa L, Perchetti GA, Phung Q, et al. A SARS-CoV-2 nucleocapsid variant that affects antigen test performance. J Clin Virol 2021;141:104900.

92. Jones TC, Biele G, Mühlemann B, et al. Estimating infectiousness throughout SARS-CoV-2 infection course. Science 2021;373(6551):eabi5273.

93. Viral infection and transmission in a large well-traced outbreak caused by the Delta SARS-CoV-2 variant - SARS-CoV-2 coronavirus/nCoV-2019 Genomic Epidemiology. Virological. 2021. Available at: https://virological.org/t/viral-infection-and-transmission-in-a-large-well-traced-outbreak-caused-by-the-delta-sars-cov-2-variant/724. Accessed October 4, 2021.

94. Lopez Bernal J, Andrews N, Gower C, et al. Effectiveness of Covid-19 Vaccines against the B.1.617.2 (Delta) variant. N Engl J Med 2021;385(7):585–94.

95. Brown CM, Vostok J, Johnson H, et al. Outbreak of SARS-CoV-2 infections, including COVID-19 vaccine breakthrough infections, associated with large public gatherings - Barnstable County, Massachusetts, July 2021. MMWR Morb Mortal Wkly Rep 2021;70(31):1059–62.

96. Shamier MC, Tostmann A, Bogers S, et al. Virological Characteristics of SARS-CoV-2 Vaccine Breakthrough Infections in Health Care Worker. doi:10.1101/2021.08.20.21262158

97. Lauren Weber and Hannah Recht RP. Many states keep patchy data or don't release results from antigen COVID tests, review shows. USA TODAY. Available at: https://www.usatoday.com/story/news/health/2020/09/16/antigen-tests-covid-19-some-states-dont-count-release-data/5806287002/. Accessed October 4, 2021.

98. Oude Munnink BB, Worp N, Nieuwenhuijse DF, et al. The next phase of SARS-CoV-2 surveillance: real-time molecular epidemiology. Nat Med 2021;27(9): 1518–24.

99. U.S. Department of Health & Human Services. COVIDtests.gov - free at-home COVID-19 tests. COVIDtests.gov. Available at: https://www.covidtests.gov/. Accessed February 14, 2022.

Clinical Diagnostic Point-of-Care Molecular Assays for SARS-CoV-2

Nicole V. Tolan, PhD, DABCC[a],*, Gary L. Horowitz, MD[b]

KEYWORDS

- Rapid nucleic acid amplification tests (NAATs) • Point-of-care testing
- COVID-19 pandemic • SARS-CoV-2 molecular assays • Method validation

KEY POINTS

- Several rapid, reliable point-of-care (POC) SARS-CoV-2 NAATs are available that provide rapid TATs with analytical performance comparable to traditional methods.
- Validation of POC methods must be done to ensure manufacturer performance specifications for the specific specimen collection and sample handling workflow implemented.
- Rapid POC SARS-CoV-2 NAATs represent a critical piece of the management of the pandemic, both at the POC but also to supplement in-laboratory testing.

INTRODUCTION

The coronavirus disease 2019 (COVID-19) pandemic presented clinical laboratories with significant challenges in meeting the demands for molecular testing. These included: (1) the inability to implement laboratory-developed nucleic acid amplification tests (NAATs) during the state of emergency, (2) managing perpetual delays in the availability of Food and Drug Administration (FDA) emergency use authorization (EUA)-cleared assays due to supply-chain issues/reagent allocations, (3) the requirement to perform unprecedented volumes of molecular tests, and (4) all while meeting the expectation that turn-around-time (TAT) become increasingly short as the pandemic proceeded. When conventional severe acute respiratory syndrome coronavirus 2 (SARS-CoV-2) NAATs became available to clinical laboratories beyond the Centers for Disease Control and Prevention (CDC) and state-run facilities, it helped address the overall demand for testing in the health care setting. However, it quickly became apparent that these traditional testing formats could not meet one particular,

[a] Department of Pathology, Brigham and Women's Hospital, Harvard Medical School, 75 Francis Street, Cotran 2, Boston, MA 01752, USA; [b] Department of Pathology and Laboratory Medicine, Tufts Medical Center, Tufts University School of Medicine, 800 Washington Street, Boston, MA 02111, USA
* Corresponding author.
E-mail address: ntolan@bwh.harvard.edu
Twitter: @NVTolan (N.V.T.)

Clin Lab Med 42 (2022) 223–236
https://doi.org/10.1016/j.cll.2022.03.002
0272-2712/22/© 2022 Elsevier Inc. All rights reserved.

labmed.theclinics.com

and very important, aspect of the demand—the need for rapid TATs for specific patient groups. Such groups include urgent care and emergency room patients with respiratory symptoms compatible with SARS-CoV-2, expectant mothers in active labor, patients who had recovered from infection and were awaiting discharge to skilled nursing facilities or other congregant living settings, and patients of all types who needed to be admitted to hospitals or undergo a potential aerosol-generating procedure (eg, intubation) to ensure they did not infect staff or other patients. Although many institutions were able to implement workflow strategies to overcome the delays of conventional SARS-CoV-2 testing (eg, testing patients 72 hours before planned procedures), inevitably, these workflows would need to be supplemented by the addition of rapid molecular testing options. Point-of-care (POC) testing offered a solution, but it required careful implementation to ensure it was fit-for-purpose. Here, we present our experience implementing rapid POC SARS-CoV-2 NAATs for clinical diagnostic testing at the Brigham and Women's Hospital (BWH) and Tufts Medical Center (Tufts) in Boston, MA, to highlight strategies used by laboratories to maintain and expand the diagnostic testing services that have been critical for rapidly identifying cases and preventing further spread of the virus.

Traditional Molecular Assays

Before the SARS-CoV-2 pandemic, most clinical laboratories were performing NAATs with conventional polymerase chain reaction (PCR) and reverse-transcriptase PCR (RT-PCR) assays. Examples include HIV and HCV viral loads, and HPV qualitative testing. These assays are FDA-cleared as Clinical Laboratory Improvement Amendments (CLIA) moderately/highly complex assays or laboratory-developed tests (LDTs) running on expensive laboratory-based instrumentation. They all have in common a TAT of several hours but are capable of testing large numbers of samples in that time frame. In the early stages of the pandemic, the laboratory-based SARS-CoV-2 NAATs developed by manufacturers were designed in similar fashion to these traditional molecular assays. A College of American Pathologists (CAP) SARS-CoV-2 proficiency testing (PT) survey from 2020 revealed that 93% of assays in use (13/14) at the time had analytical times that did not meet the requirements for rapid molecular testing.

POC NAATs for other respiratory viruses such as influenza A/B (Flu) and respiratory syncytial virus (RSV) have been commercially available for several years. These platforms are capable of providing rapid TAT results albeit with low throughput, and many are also CLIA-waived, which allows them to be performed in clinical settings by non–laboratory-trained individuals such as nurses and medical assistants. As the pandemic proceeded, these platforms were expanded to diagnose SARS-CoV-2 alone or as a multiplex panel, thus offering a pathway for using rapid molecular results in select patient populations. Accordingly, a significant increase was observed in the number of laboratories using rapid NAAT platforms as their primary method for SARS-CoV-2 diagnostics, from 680 in the 2020 CAP survey to 2739 laboratories in 2021. This is likely an underestimate given that CLIA-waived devices do not formally require participation in a PT program. There is a clear use case for many laboratories to supplement their large laboratory equipment with these single-use, cartridge-based methods within the laboratory itself.

Rapid SARS-CoV-2 NAAT POC Methods

Manufacturers developed SARS-CoV-2 NAATs for systems that were already on the market, with the major examples being the Abbott ID NOW COVID-19,[1] the Cepheid GeneXpert Xpress SARS-CoV-2,[2] and the Roche LIAT.[3] These methods leveraged existing technologies, and either substituted the primer-probe sets with those specific to SARS-CoV-2 or added them to the influenza/RSV sets to offer a respiratory virus panel. As detailed in **Table 1**, these methods are classified as rapid molecular assays that incorporate either traditional RT-PCR or isothermal nucleic acid amplification and are capable of producing results in less than 60 min. They are cartridge-based methods that incorporate the reagents necessary for amplification of the complementary DNA template of the viral RNA contained within the respiratory sample as well as an internal control to ensure against false-negative results with assay malfunctions. These methods have predominately targeted the RNA-dependent RNA polymerase (RdRP), nucleocapsid N2, and envelope E genes. They have been approved for use in laboratories with high- (H) and moderate- (M) CLIA certificates as well as patient care settings operating under a CLIA Certificate of Waiver (W). Throughout the pandemic, these assays have been available as SARS-CoV-2 only tests but 2 of the 3 major manufacturers we highlight have also incorporated other targets to create a respiratory panel test.

An interesting approach to providing rapid and inexpensive NAATs for SARS-CoV-2 detection at the POC has been the adaptation of reverse transcription loop-mediated isothermal amplification (RT-LAMP) technology.[4,5] In contrast to conventional RT-PCR, which requires multiple cycles of heating and cooling (thermocycling) to amplify target RNA (**Fig. 1**A), LAMP assays are isothermal. RT-LAMP significantly reduces the amplification time typically required for thermocycling of the primers that extend the DNA template (**Fig. 1**B). Typical RT-LAMP assays can be completed in under an hour, and in some cases as quickly as 15 minutes. One commercial assay, the Lucira CHECK-IT COVID-19 Test Kit,[6] received FDA EUA for home use with a physician's order and then later, for over-the-counter (OTC) and direct-to-consumer (DTC) use. This method can provide positive results in as little as 11 minutes; however, it has yet to be widely adopted for clinical diagnostic use because of concerns over sensitivity compared to traditional RT-PCR.[7–9]

Validation

In most US states, tests categorized as CLIA-waived do not require local laboratory validation; they can be used based entirely on the data submitted to the FDA for

Table 1
CLIA-waived POC SARS-CoV-2 molecular assays predominately used in the hospital setting

Entity, Diagnostic	Date of EUA	Attributes	Authorized Settings
Abbott ID NOW SARS-CoV-2	03/27/2020	RT, Isothermal amplification ($\leq$13 min)	H,M,W
Cepheid Xpert Xpress SARS-CoV-2	03/20/2020	Real-time RT-PCR (56 min)	H,M,W
SARS-CoV-2/Flu/RSV	09/24/2020	Multi-Analyte (38 min)	H,M,W
Roche LIAT SARS-CoV-2	6/17/2021	Real-time RT-PCR ($\sim$20 min)	H,M,W
SARS-CoV-2/Flu	9/14/2020	Multi-Analyte ($\sim$20 min)	H,M,W

Abbreviations: H, high-complexity testing; M, moderate-complexity testing; W, patient care settings operating under a CLIA Certificate of Waiver.
Summarized from: https://www.fda.gov/medical-devices/coronavirus-disease-2019-covid-19-emergency-use-authorizations-medical-devices/in-vitro-diagnostics-euas-molecular-diagnostic-tests-sars-cov-2#individual-molecular, Accessed: 07/01/2021

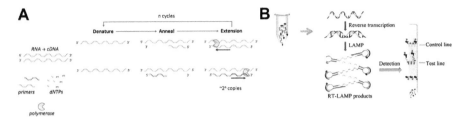

Fig. 1. Comparison of the mechanism of (*A*) traditional RT-PCR requiring 3 to 5 hours and thermocycling equipment to (*B*) RT-LAMP technology requiring 10 to 60 minutes performed isothermally. (*A*) Author's Original; (*B*) *Adapted from* Huang et al[4] with permission from Frontiers in Microbiology (2018).

ensuring the test performance characteristics. These methods have been determined by the FDA as simple to perform and have low risk for erroneous results. To maintain this distinction, sites using CLIA-waived tests must strictly follow all of the manufacturer's instructions. Simply put, this classification allows sites with a CLIA waiver to simply plug in the device, train the operators, and follow the instructions to perform patient testing. However, in our experience, this system of FDA review does not necessarily ensure that performance expectations are met when deployed for clinical diagnostic testing, particularly during a crisis on the scale of the COVID-19 pandemic.

Although certain states do not require formal validation studies for CLIA-waived tests, many laboratories still choose to perform validations. The POC SARS-CoV-2 NAATs implemented in clinical laboratories in the United States, just like the CLIA moderately and highly complex counterparts, were EUA-cleared as qualitative tests, which simplifies the validation studies. When reporting qualitatively, the validation of sample precision, accuracy, analytical specificity, and sensitivity are the major focus. Sample precision, or repeatability through replicate testing, typically requires samples with known concentrations—either patient samples with quantitative results determined by a reference method, quality control (QC) material, or calibration standards with assigned values. Ideally, these should be a mix of positive and negative samples near the threshold and not simply at either extreme of the assay results. Accuracy studies are performed to demonstrate the qualitative comparability of results to a reference method. Without knowing the viral copy number or cycle threshold (Ct) values of the positive samples of the samples included in the validation, it would be quite possible for laboratories to miss differences in performance. As shown in **Fig. 2**A, the qualitative comparison of the Roche LIAT was performed against the laboratory-based Panther Fusion and Cepheid GeneXpert methods. Here, 28 residual frozen samples were selected over a wide range of Ct values, which are inversely proportional to viral copy numbers. Only a single sample with an original Ct value of 39, near the positive threshold of 42 on the Panther Fusion, was found to be negative after thawing and running by LIAT. The sample was repeated on the Cepheid GeneXpert and was confirmed to be negative. The analytical specificity, or interference, can largely be inferred from the manufacturer's FDA submission studies and peer-reviewed literature. For the LIAT validation, 10 SARS-CoV-2 negative samples that were positive for commonly circulating pathogens were evaluated and were shown be to 100% concordant with the reference methods.

As it pertains to SARS-CoV-2, many health care providers and infection control specialists have found utility in reviewing Ct values to differentiate patients with high viral loads from those who have a small amount of residual RNA remaining in the setting of resolved infection.[10,11] The reporting of Ct values is considered a modification of the

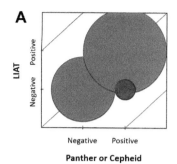

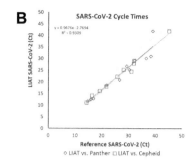

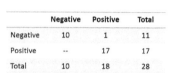

	Negative	Positive	Total
Negative	10	1	11
Positive	--	17	17
Total	10	18	28

	Panther	GeneXpert
Deming Regression	y=1.052x-5.06	y=1.007-3.80
	R=0.9586	R=0.9919
Bias (%)	-3.62 (-13.19%)	-3.35 (-12.63%)

Fig. 2. SARS-CoV-2 LIAT accuracy validation against the traditional Panther Fusion and Cepheid GeneXpert NAAT methods for (*A*) qualitative and (*B*) quantitative reporting of cycle time (Ct value).

EUA-cleared method and requires additional validation of quantitative precision to ensure reproducible results and verifying the comparability between methods. Studies for quantitative interassay (between day) precision are typically conducted using QC material, as outlined earlier, with Ct values at multiple points throughout the reportable range to ensure the variability (measured as the coefficient of variation) is clinically acceptable. With respect to quantitative accuracy, **Fig. 2**B shows excellent correlation in Ct values between the LIAT method and the 2 reference methods that were clinically available at the time, the Panther Fusion and Cepheid GeneXpert. There was a minor systematic bias as the LIAT method is shown to run, on average, 3.5 cycles (12.9%) lower, which is consistent with findings reported in a 2020 letter to the editor of *Clinical Infectious Disease,* in which the CAP Microbiology Committee warned of the risks of interpreting Ct values of SARS-CoV-2 molecular assays.[12] However, aside from the Abbott m2000, the remaining 7 methods analyzed in the letter had median Ct results with relatively good agreement using the same batch of PT material, across multiple manufacturers' methods and various gene targets. Therefore, it would seem reasonable to be able to use this datum to reliably differentiate high versus low Ct values in the clinical context of a given patient's presentation. However, the Ct ranges observed for patients without symptomatic disease or with low levels of virus require additional studies beyond those currently available[12–14]; the details of which are beyond the scope of this article. Regardless, if a laboratory were to choose to report Ct values, the comparability across clinically reported methods must be evaluated and the results accompanied by sufficient interpretation, by way of automatic result comments or other means of appropriately interpretive comments.

Beyond these components of the validation, even for qualitatively reported assays, it is particularly important to verify the manufacturer's claims of performance in terms of the analytical sensitivity and limit of detection (LOD). The traditional method of assessing the analytical sensitivity of NAATs is to prepare a series of reference standard dilutions, which are then run in replicate. The conventional definition of the LOD represents the lowest concentration that can be detected at least 95% of the time (eg, 20 of 21 replicates). Most laboratories cannot run such extensive numbers of replicates, but they can make a reasonable assessment of the LOD with fewer replicates. As shown in **Fig. 3**A, multiple dilutions of a SARS-CoV-2 standard (5336 copies/mL, AccuPlex SARS-CoV-2 Reference Material, SeraCare, Milford, MA) confirmed that the Cepheid assay detected concentrations down to roughly 60 copies/mL. An alternative approach to determining analytical sensitivity, which is perhaps more informative, is to compare clinical specimens against a previously validated, highly sensitive comparison method. As shown in the top panel of **Fig. 3**B, 47 patient samples with estimated copy numbers (log copies/mL) determined using the Abbott m2000 were evaluated by the Cepheid Xpert Xpress, which in this case is the "test" method. The LOD of the Abbott m2000 method had previously been formally confirmed using a reference standard, as described earlier. With this set of clinical specimens, the lowest positive concentration that the Cepheid could determine (ie, with no false-negative results) was approximately 80 copies/mL, which was roughly equivalent to the previous study using the externally purchased standard material. Examples of similar comparisons of 2 other SARS-CoV-2 NAATs are reflected for an LDT method (**Fig. 3**C) and a traditional NAAT (**Fig. 3**D). Neither of these could reliably detect concentrations as low as the Cepheid, with their cut-off limits being roughly 180 and 8500 copies/mL, respectively.

In the absence of a standard curve relating Ct values to viral RNA copy numbers, many studies were reported comparing positive and negative percent agreements (PPA and NPA) with highly sensitive NAATs, the method required by the FDA EUA authorization template for molecular tests.[15,16] These reports used a wide range of comparator methods and patient populations, but they still provide useful information. **Table 2** shows a compilation of the data from a meta-analysis of the ID NOW,[17] indicating that it has excellent NPA but a suboptimal PPA of approximately 70% (with 30% false-negative results).

An interesting aspect of the Lucira package insert is that it provided clinical performance data as a function of viral RNA concentration.[6] In 2 studies in community

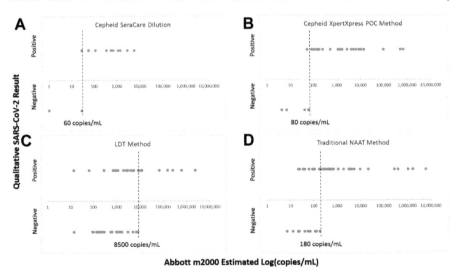

Fig. 3. Analytical sensitivity determination using (*A*) a standard with known viral copy numbers (SeraCare: 5663 copies/mL) and (*B–D*) three sets of real patient samples as compared to the estimated copy numbers determined by a highly-sensitive reference method, Abbott m2000, for 3 SARS-CoV-2 NAAT methods. The limit of detection is shown for each method by the dashed vertical line.

Table 2
Summary of meta-analysis for the reported performance of the Abbott ID NOW SARS-CoV-2 method

Study #	TP	FN	FP	TN	Total	PPA (%)	NPA (%)
1	12	15	0	60	87	44.4	100.0
2	17	14	1	69	101	54.8	98.6
3	12	1	0	169	182	92.3	100.0
4	139	47	2	336	524	74.7	99.4
5	4	2	0	46	52	66.7	100.0
6	33	13	0	15	61	71.7	100.0
7	94	31	0	73	198	75.2	100.0
8	90	6	0	0	96	93.8	UTC
9	65	23	0	25	113	73.9	100.0
10	8	7	0	167	182	53.3	100.0
11	50	7	0	50	107	87.7	100.0
12	0	1	0	116	117	0.0	100.0
13	16	1	1	95	113	94.1	99.0
14	23	0	0	35	58	100.0	100.0
Total	563	168	4	1256	1991	77.0	99.7

Abbreviations: FN, false negative; FP, false positive; NPA, negative percent agreement; PPA, positive percent agreement; TN, true negative; TP, true positive; UTC, unable to calculate.

Summarized from Tu et al. eLife 2021; 10:e65726. DOI: https://doi.org/10.7554/eLife.65726. Accessed: 07/01/2021

settings, the Lucira NAAT showed an overall PPA of 92% on 404 specimens from symptomatic and asymptomatic patients, including 10 specimens with very low viral RNA concentrations. Excluding these specimens, whose Ct values were greater than 37.5, the assay was shown to be 98% accurate in comparison to high-sensitivity laboratory assays.

The ability to maintain a single sample type was challenging throughout the pandemic without reliable sources of collection swabs and transport media. Furthermore, experts were concerned about the loss of sensitivity as samples deviated from the preferred nasopharyngeal (NP) swabs. In addition to traditional NP swabs, 3 major POC methods used in clinical laboratories did receive EUA for some combination of anterior nares (nasal) swabs, nasal midturbinate, oropharyngeal, and in some cases, nasal wash/aspirate collection types. A few studies have also suggested reliable results from alternate specimen types including oral fluid,[18] stool, and ocular secretions,[19,20] but outside of saliva, these are not in widespread use. To ensure comparability in method performance across sample types, it is essential for laboratories to separately validate alternate collection materials/conditions, with a particular focus on specimens with low viral RNA copy numbers.

Implementation

The actual implementation of assays categorized by the FDA as waived and designed to be performed at the POC requires additional considerations beyond assay performance.

Assays that are CLIA-waived have a major advantage in that they have reduced educational requirements for the testing personnel and can be performed by laboratory accessioning staff, medical assistants, nurses, and other nontechnical staff. This offers the opportunity for implementing these assays within the clinical laboratory itself for triaging specimens with rapid TAT requests, but without requiring the same technologists who meet the educational requirements of moderate- and high-complexity testing. Furthermore, although federal CLIA and state requirements apply whether performing the test in the laboratory or truly at the POC, the laboratory setting is much more conducive to the rigorous laboratory quality essentials as compared with the clinical settings like the emergency department, which are staffed by personnel focused on patient care.

When one considers the workflows affecting the TAT of NAATs used in the laboratory setting, one needs to take into account many factors beyond the analytical time of the assay. These include the time required for:

- Preparing the specimen for transport to the laboratory
- Transporting the specimen, often in a batched process
- Receiving and/or accessioning the specimen into the laboratory information system
- Preanalytical processing, which depends on the NAAT used
- Resulting and transmitting the result to the ordering provider and clinical team.

If the analytical time is measured in hours, these other factors may represent a relatively small fraction of the overall TAT. However, when they are all combined, they lead to significant additional delays compared with implementing these rapid methods at the POC (**Fig. 4**). Although POC NAATs cannot compete with traditional NAATs within the laboratory, in terms of providing high-throughput testing volumes on a daily basis, they can outperform these tests in providing reliable, actionable results within minutes to an hour of specimen collection (depending on the workflow). In the best-case scenario, sample transport and receipt into the laboratory would be limited to 1 hour, there would be no batching delays and specimens would be tested as they were received, analytical times would be no longer than 2 hours and the instrument would be interfaced with results reporting into the electronic record without significant delay in the provider reviewing the results. With these parameters, the laboratory testing workflow could be as short as 3 hours from the time of collection (see **Fig. 4**). However, this certainly is not the case for all clinical laboratories and may not even be consistent throughout the week, or even a given day (**Fig. 5**). Therefore, from a purely TAT standpoint, implementing POC rapid NAATs in the clinic at the point of specimen collection, rather than the laboratory, reduces the TAT to less than 60 min and is mostly reliant on the analytical time of the method.

POC tests can be performed by operators with limited laboratory skills as compared with the highly trained and qualified laboratory personnel required for most traditional NAATs. Indeed, the same person collecting the specimen can run the test, while wearing the same personal protective equipment. To protect staff, laboratories that perform infectious disease testing, whether it be culture or NAAT, often use biologic hoods for specimen preparation. However, for SARS-CoV-2 testing, the use of biologic hoods is not required by the EUAs covering POC NAATs. Arguably, the greatest risk of acquiring SARS-CoV-2 for staff at the POC relates more to their direct interactions with patients, and specifically specimen acquisition, as opposed to specimen processing on the assay. Thus, the personal protective equipment requirements for specimen collection are sufficient for testing personnel to guard against any potential aerosolizing steps (eg, vortexing) of the testing procedure.

We took advantage of a number of these aspects at our respective institutions. At BWH, LIATs were deployed in the microbiology laboratory, as well as in the laboratory

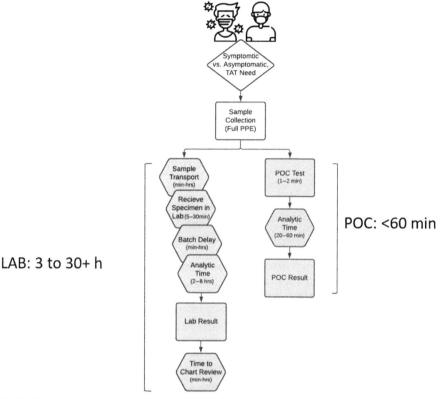

Fig. 4. Comparison of SARS-CoV-2 laboratory-based testing with the POC workflow. Traditional laboratory-based workflows typically incur delays from (1) sample transport, (2) batch delays, and (3) longer analytical time as compared with POC workflows requiring less than 60 minutes and are highly dependent on analytical assay time, which is much shorter.

of an affiliate urgent care clinic, separate from the main hospital. Although not truly implemented at the POC, the laboratories found great value in offering this rapid, cartridge-based method to meet the TAT needs of hospital-based urgent testing (eg, asymptomatic patients presenting to the ED, preprocedural, admit/discharge) and reduce the time for results from the off-site urgent care clinic testing symptomatic patients, that would otherwise incur long-delays in batched transport back to the main campus laboratory. This workflow allowed the laboratory to provide a TAT of approximately 1 hour from sample collection by reducing the analytical time to approximately 20 min on the Roche LIAT (see **Table 1**). At Tufts, LIATs and GeneXpert methods were deployed in the central laboratory to achieve the same goal, and the use of these methods was not restricted to just patients in the emergency room, but was expanded, as reagent supplies allowed, to any patient for whom the infectious diseases consulting physicians needed rapid results. In addition, LIATs were deployed as genuine POC devices at 4 individual affiliated urgent care sites, where results were reported in real-time. The total test volumes peaked at roughly 600 per week and often exceeded the volumes of rapid NAATs performed by the laboratory (approximately 250 per week), indicating that they were providing an extremely valuable service in the communities they served.

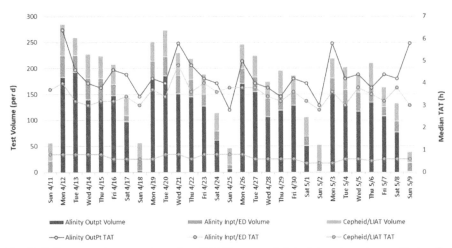

Fig. 5. Daily test volume and median TAT (from receipt in laboratory to result) for the laboratory-based Abbott Alinity method (2-hour analytical time, used for outpatient and inpatient/ED) and Cepheid/LIAT POCT assays performed at Tufts Medical Center. TAT goals were established as: Alinity outpatient: ≤6 hours; Alinity inpatient/ED: ≤4 hours; and Cepheid/LIAT: ≤1 hour.

As previously discussed, attention to specimen types and specimen acquisition is important for all SARS-CoV-2 NAATs. However, this deserves special emphasis for POC testing, where nontechnical staff perform the tests and may be less vigilant about observing requirements. Only the types of specimens covered by the EUA and validated by the laboratory should be processed. Early in the pandemic, only properly collected NP swabs could be used. Midturbinate, anterior nasal, and other specimen types were easier to collect but represented different matrices and likely had different nucleic acid concentrations depending on where the individual was on their viral replication curve. As these other specimen types were added to POC EUAs, they could be used but required in-house validation and clear communication to clinicians as to the potential for reduced performance (see above).

Once collected, specimen handling issues become paramount. Whether testing is performed at the POC or in a traditional laboratory, appropriate labeling of specimens is critical, but the temptation to be more lax with this requirement is far greater at the POC. In most cases, specimen swabs have to be placed in viral transport media, at which point specimen stability for testing is assured for suitable lengths of time. In some cases, however, specimens need to be tested directly within an hour of collection (eg, Abbott IDNOW). In all cases, the testing process must follow the manufacturer's instructions and laboratory validated protocols to remain unmodified and CLIA-waived.

Once testing is complete, it is critical not only to inform the patient's caregivers but also to enter the results into the medical record and to report them to local public health authorities. One of the advantages of POC testing is that informing the patient's caregivers is usually straightforward, especially if the testing is completed while the patient and caregivers are still present. But it is critically important that the information be accurately captured in the medical record, particularly for patient precautions, but to also ensure reporting to public health authorities. Many of the POC devices are capable of being interfaced with laboratory information systems, a feature whose importance should not be understated. The effort required to build and maintain this interface must also not be underestimated. Manual transcription of results is not as reliable and requires error-checking for accuracy, something that can be challenging to enforce at the POC, particularly when testing volumes are high. As compared with other POC methods (eg, rapid Streptococcal antigen tests), relying on a physician's note to capture SARS-CoV-2 NAAT results severely limits the ability to interface with state reporting mechanisms, challenges the ability for local institution tracking, and managing patient precautions for the safety of other healthcare providers.

Beyond the qualitative result reporting, simply as "positive" or "negative" (or "detected" or "not detected"), the assay performance limitations must be communicated to the ordering provider. At the onset of COVID-19, clear statements of assay limitations were required by the EUA to include disclaimers indicating, for example, that negative results do not preclude SARS-CoV-2 infections and should not be used as the sole basis for treatment or other patient management decisions. As time progressed, these statements of limitations were maintained in the EUA but there were no longer requirements for this disclaimer to accompany each result report in the medical record. However, clear understanding and communication of assay performance differences remain.

DISCUSSION

During the initial phases of the COVID-19 pandemic, it was widely recognized that unprecedented numbers of NAATs needed to be performed to monitor and control the spread of the virus. Traditional RT-PCR assays were well suited to addressing this need, with individual instruments capable of performing thousands of tests per day. Even so, demand far surpassed capacity. Clinically significant delays in reporting results (often exceeding 1–2 days and sometimes as long as 5–7 days) occurred at clinical laboratories, public health laboratories, and ultimately even at large commercial laboratories. These delays caused by demand were soon exacerbated by reagent and other supply shortages. As important as it was to provide large numbers of reliable results, there was also a need to deliver faster TATs to manage certain populations of patients, particularly those in urgent care settings and emergency rooms who would require admission to hospitals to determine bed placement and precautions for staff. This was a niche that could be filled extremely well by POC rapid NAATs. The analytical times, almost always less than an hour, were the most attractive aspect of this strategy. One downside of these assays is throughput, which can be made mitigated by limiting testing to those patients who need it most.

In our experience, the analytical sensitivity of POC NAATs is often adequate and in some cases, even better than some conventional laboratory-based RT-PCR NAATs. However, it is critical that they be validated by the laboratory rather than rely solely on manufacturer data. Although the FDA template for EUA for these POC CLIA-waived assays mandated comparison to highly sensitive methods, it did not prescribe that a range of viral concentrations be included in those assessments. Because of differences in the comparison method used, in the populations tested, and in the specimen types used, the NPA and PPA might be excellent even for an assay with less than optimal analytical sensitivity. As one example, the Abbott ID NOW assay was determined by many independent investigators to have lower sensitivity than other NAATs, with differences large enough to be potentially clinically significant. Abbott ultimately updated the ID NOW package insert, indicating that tests could only be done in patients whose symptoms were compatible with COVID-19 and within 7 days of symptom onset, the time frame when viral concentrations in upper respiratory specimens are highest. This does not suggest that the ID NOW is a poor test. Rather, it means its use should be limited to patients who meet their defined criteria for testing.[17,21]

With respect to implementation, several aspects of CLIA-waived POC rapid NAATs should be noted. The first is the reduced educational requirements for testing personnel, allowing the tests to be performed by nontechnical staff within the laboratory and at the POC. As a result, workflows can be optimized, allowing for TATs of less than an hour from specimen collection. Second, especially at sites outside the laboratory, vigilance is required in maintaining adherence to specimen types and specimen handling. The third is the importance of capturing results in the medical record and transmitting them to public health authorities, requiring sufficient support and resources to implement and maintain electronic interfacing.

One of the more interesting aspects of POC SARS-CoV-2 NAATs is their costs. In general, the actual cost to produce results with a POC test is far more than the cost to do the same test in the central laboratory. This is often related to the reagent costs and inability to leverage economies of scale like in large central laboratories, as well as incremental labor and capital equipment costs. It was our experience that the costs associated with POC SARS-CoV-2 NAATs were often comparable to their laboratory-based counterparts, unless one pooled specimens or developed one's own assay, which the overwhelming majority of laboratories did not do. Regardless, even if POC NAATs clearly did cost more, their beneficial impact in terms of added safety to the patient, staff, and other patients in hospitals and residents in community living settings arguably more than offset those costs.

It is important to point out that rapid POC NAATs existed prepandemic. A particularly good example is for influenza testing. At a time when rapid antigen tests were not sensitive enough to reliably rule out influenza, it was strongly suggested that all negative tests performed at the POC be confirmed by NAAT. As most tests were negative, this translated into excessive delays to get definitive results on most specimens with additive costs for both assays. POC NAATs for flu provided an excellent solution to the problem and enhanced patient care, providing real-time patient-physician interaction and ability to prescribe antiviral medication when indicated. Looking to the future, one wonders whether we can provide POC NAATs for other diseases, like HIV or HCV, where many patients are lost to follow-up before they can be connected to care.[22]

In summary, POC SARS-CoV-2 NAATs, properly validated and implemented, represent extremely valuable resources, for POC sites as well as traditional laboratories. They should not be seen, as many POC assays are, as inferior and more expensive counterparts to moderately and highly complex traditional laboratory assays. Central laboratories can, and should, assist with validating and implementing these assays, helping to ensure they are fit for purpose. In doing so, they may find that these assays can play a vital role in addressing their own needs for reliable, appropriately sensitive, rapid turnaround time assays. POC SARS-CoV-2 NAATs represent another example of the continuum of laboratory testing, and it is vital that traditional laboratories embrace them in helping us meet our role in delivering the highest level of quality patient care.

CLINICS CARE POINTS

- Although certain states do not require formal validation of CLIA-waived POC SARS-CoV-2 NAATs, it is highly recommended that laboratories evaluate the method performance.
  - Even when reporting results qualitatively, it is particularly important to determine the limit of detection/analytical sensitivity using specimens with known cycle threshold (Ct) values that span the clinical range.

- Additional considerations exist if Ct values are made available to treating clinicians, including the need to:
  - Determine assay precision (variability within sample)
  - Perform method comparison (variability across methods)
  - Establish the clinical acceptability of the assay for differentiating very low viral copies (residual RNA) from high copies (acute infection, increasing over time)
- POCT methods offer several advantages but implementation and regulatory compliance can be challenging.
  - CLIA-waived methods have reduced educational requirements for operators and can be run by non–laboratory-trained staff.
  - Although not well-suited for high-throughput demands, POC SARS-CoV-2 NAATs can offer rapid TAT at the POC but also when implemented within-laboratory.
  - It can be particularly challenging to maintain compliance with assay and regulatory requirements at the POC, particularly with regards to:
    - Staying within the clinical indications of use (eg, including testing only symptomatic individuals, and/or within a certain number of days since symptom onset)
    - Testing only approved specimen types and following sample handling requirements
    - Communication of assay limitations to treating clinicians and maintaining state/federal reporting requirements

DISCLOSURE

The authors have nothing to disclose.

ACKNOWLEDGMENTS

Dedicated laboratory professionals supporting patient testing throughout the COVID-19 pandemic.

REFERENCES

1. Abbott diagnostics ID NOW COVID-19 instructions for Use (Rev. 7 2020/09). Available at: https://www.fda.gov/media/136525/download. Accessed July 1, 2021.
2. Cepheid Xpert Xpress SARS-CoV-2 instructions for Use (Rev. F January 2021). Available at: https://www.fda.gov/media/136315/download. Accessed July 1, 2021.
3. Roche molecular systems cobas SARS-CoV-2 & influenza A/B nucleic acid test instructions for Use (Rev. 2.0). Available at: https://www.fda.gov/media/142193/download. Accessed July 1, 2021.
4. Huang P, Wang H, Cao Z, et al. A rapid and specific assay for the detection of MERS-CoV. Front Microbiol 2018;9:1101.
5. Ganguli A, Mostafa A, Berger J, et al. Rapid Isothermal Amplification and Portable Detection System for SARS-CoV-2. bioRxiv : the preprint server for biology. 2020.
6. Lucira health CHECK-IT COVID-19 test Kit instructions for Use (INST017 Rev. 4). Available at: https://www.fda.gov/media/147495/download. Accessed July 1, 2021.
7. Schellenberg JJ, Ormond M, Keynan Y. Extraction-free RT-LAMP to detect SARS-CoV-2 is less sensitive but highly specific compared to standard RT-PCR in 101 samples. J Clin Virol 2021;136:104764.
8. de Oliveira Coelho B, Sanchuki HBS, Zanette DL, et al. Essential properties and pitfalls of colorimetric Reverse Transcription Loop-mediated Isothermal Amplification as a point-of-care test for SARS-CoV-2 diagnosis. Mol Med 2021;27(1):30.

9. Wang R, Qian C, Pang Y, et al. opvCRISPR: one-pot visual RT-LAMP-CRISPR platform for SARS-cov-2 detection. Biosens Bioelectron 2021;172:112766.

10. Tom MR, Mina MJ. To Interpret the SARS-CoV-2 test, consider the cycle threshold value. Clin Infect Dis 2020;71(16):2252–4.

11. Binnicker MJ. Can the severe acute respiratory syndrome coronavirus 2 polymerase Chain reaction cycle threshold value and time from symptom onset to testing predict infectivity? Clin Infect Dis 2020;71(10):2667–8.

12. Rhoads D, Peaper DR, She RC, et al. College of American Pathologists (CAP) microbiology Committee Perspective: Caution must Be used in interpreting the cycle threshold (Ct) value. Clin Infect Dis 2021;72(10):e685–6.

13. Bullard J, Dust K, Funk D, et al. Predicting infectious severe acute respiratory syndrome coronavirus 2 from diagnostic samples. Clin Infect Dis 2020;71(10):2663–6.

14. Infectious Diseases Society of America and Association for Molecular Pathology. IDSA and AMP joint statement on the use of SARS-CoV-2 PCR cycle threshold (Ct) values for clinical decision-making. Updated March 12, 2021. Available at: https://www.idsociety.org/globalassets/idsa/public-health/covid-19/idsa-amp-statement.pdf. Accessed July 1, 2021.

15. Food and Drug Administration. In Vitro diagnostic emergency Use authorizations: molecular diagnostic template for commercial manufacturers (updated July 28, 2020). Available at: https://www.fda.gov/media/135900/download. Accessed July 1, 2021.

16. Food and Drug Administration. In Vitro diagnostic emergency Use authorizations: template for manufacturers of molecular and antigen diagnostic COVID-19 tests for non-laboratory Use (July 29, 2020). Available at: https://www.fda.gov/media/140615/download. Accessed July 1, 2021.

17. Tu YP, Iqbal J, O'Leary T. Sensitivity of ID NOW and RT-PCR for detection of SARS-CoV-2 in an ambulatory population. eLife 2021;10:e65726.

18. Vogels CBF, Watkins AE, Harden CA, et al. SalivaDirect: a simplified and flexible platform to enhance SARS-CoV-2 testing capacity. Med (N Y) 2021;2(3):263–80.e6.

19. Xia J, Tong J, Liu M, et al. Evaluation of coronavirus in tears and conjunctival secretions of patients with SARS-CoV-2 infection. J Med Virol 2020;92(6):589–94.

20. COVID-19 Investigation Team. Clinical and virologic characteristics of the first 12 patients with coronavirus disease 2019 (COVID-19) in the United States. Nat Med 2020;26(6):861–8.

21. Abbott Releases ID NOW™ COVID-19 Interim Clinical Study Results from 1,003 People to Provide the Facts on Clinical Performance and to Support Public Health. PR Newswire: Cision

22. Tolan NV, Horowitz GL, Graham CS, et al. New therapies for treating hepatitis c virus: impact on laboratory testing recommendations and clinical management. Clin Chem 2017;63(12):1799–805.

Cycle Threshold Values from Severe Acute Respiratory Syndrome Coronavirus-2 Reverse Transcription-Polymerase Chain Reaction Assays

Interpretation and Potential Use Cases

Alexander J. McAdam, MD, PhD

KEYWORDS

- COVID-19 • SARS-CoV-2 • Reverse transcription-polymerase chain reaction
- Cycle threshold value

KEY POINTS

- The cycle threshold (Ct) value is a semi-quantitative value that is inversely related to the level of viral RNA in reverse transcription-polymerase chain reaction (RT-PCR) tests for severe acute respiratory syndrome coronavirus-2 (SARS-CoV-2)
- The Ct value for SARS-CoV-2 is inherently variable due to the variability of RT-PCR, and further variability can be introduced by sample factors (collection, storage, sample type), and use of different RT-PCR tests.
- Potential clinical uses of Ct values for SARS-CoV-2 include the assessment of the progression of infection, prediction of disease severity, and determination of infectivity.
- Caregivers using Ct values for these purposes must understand the variability and limitations of Ct values, which can be facilitated by direct communication with the leadership of the clinical laboratory.

INTRODUCTION

The coronavirus disease 2019 (COVID-19) pandemic, caused by the severe acute respiratory syndrome coronavirus-2 (SARS-CoV-2) has caused more than 381 million infections and more than 5.6 million deaths, worldwide, including more than 75 million infections and more than 890,000 deaths in the United States (US).[1] While the use

Infectious Diseases Diagnostic Laboratory, Department of Laboratory Medicine, Boston Children's Hospital, Harvard Medical School, 300 Longwood Avenue, Boston, MA 02115, USA
E-mail address: alexander.mcadam@childrens.harvard.edu
Twitter: @JClinMicro (A.J.M.)

Clin Lab Med 42 (2022) 237–248
https://doi.org/10.1016/j.cll.2022.02.003
0272-2712/22/© 2022 Elsevier Inc. All rights reserved.

of vaccines has slowed the mortality rates in many places, lack of access to vaccines and vaccine hesitancy has resulted in continued infections and deaths. Diagnostic testing for SARS-CoV-2 has been and will continue to be critical to addressing the pandemic.

The mainstay of diagnostic testing is nucleic acid amplified tests, primarily using reverse transcription followed by polymerase chain reaction (RT-PCR). RT-PCR tests for SARS-CoV-2 are designed and validated to be used as qualitative tests, reporting as positive if the virus is detected or negative if it is not. RT-PCR can be made quantitative if a standard curve is generated using known concentrations of virus or viral RNA, allowing the use of the sample cycle threshold (Ct) at which viral RNA is detected to estimate the quantity of virus present. Alternatively, the Ct value alone can be used directly, as a semi-quantitative way to compare the level of virus between 2 samples run using the same assay on the same platform.

While PCR and RT-PCR have been used to detect viral pathogens for several years, is it only during the COVID-19 pandemic that there has been serious consideration of using Ct values for clinical care and infection control measures. This has been an area of active debate. Professional organizations, including the Association for Molecular Pathology, Infectious Diseases Society of America, the Association of Public Health Laboratories, and the American Association of Clinical Chemistry have issued guidelines against using Ct values for clinical care.[2–4] Regardless of this, laboratory directors are frequently asked to supply Ct values for various purposes, discussed later in discussion, and need to be prepared for such requests. Furthermore, in at least one state in the US, Florida, clinical laboratories are required to report Ct values to the state Department of Public Health, but not in clinical reports to care providers.[5]

Before turning to a discussion of the potential uses of Ct values, it is important to understand the regulatory status of reporting Ct values for SARS-CoV-2. Because RT-PCRs for SARS-CoV-2 have been approved for use as qualitative assays, reporting a quantitative result, such as a Ct value, is a regulatory violation.[3] Reporting these values to providers outside of the laboratory report does not necessarily prevent them from appearing in the medical record, as they can be included in the clinical notes. Laboratory directors should understand the potential consequences of reporting Ct values and consider this in determining how and whether to provide these values for clinical care.

The remainder of this review will include 3 topics. First, the variability of Ct values for SARS-CoV-2 will be briefly discussed, as this is important to understanding the potential utility of these values. Second, the evidence for and against various uses of Ct values will be reviewed. Finally, specific recommendations will be made for those who have decided to provide Ct values to clinical caregivers or for infection control purposes.

Variability of Cycle Threshold Values

It is important to understand the sources and magnitude of variability of Ct values for SARS-CoV-2. This variability can be reduced or minimized, but it cannot be eliminated (**Table 1**). Clinical staff should understand that Ct values can be highly variable and this is one of the several reasons why these values must be interpreted with caution. Information about the variability of Ct values can be provided within the laboratory report or during consultation between the laboratory director and clinical staff, before the release of Ct values. These data should not be provided without a complete explanation of the expected variability and of what changes might be considered meaningful in the context of clinical care.

Table 1 Sources of variability in RT-PCR for SARS-CoV-2		
Source of Variability	**Magnitude of Variation**	**Mitigation Strategies**
Use of different RT-PCR Assays	Small to large	Use the same assay, performed in the same laboratory if values will be compared between different samples
Transport Media	Small	Not needed
Sample Storage	Small if samples are less than a week old at temperatures from room temperature to −80°C Moderate if samples are held longer than a week at room temperature or 4°C (low-levels of RNA may become undetectable)	If sample retention is longer than a week, freeze samples, preferably at −80C
Sample type	Small to moderate, with nasopharyngeal swabs generally having lower Ct values than other samples from the upper respiratory tract	Use the same type of sample if values are compared between samples Nasopharyngeal swab samples may be preferred if Ct values are compared

Variations in Ct values are designated as small if they are 2 or smaller, moderate if they are greater than 2 but smaller than 7, and large if they are 7 or greater.

There are several sources of variability in Ct values, and these are discussed separately in the sections that follow. In considering these sources of variability, several things should be kept in mind. First, the methods used in these studies vary significantly. For brevity, the most important differences in methods will be discussed, but less important differences will not. Second, these papers often show summary data, such as means and standard deviations, graphically, but they may not provide the numerical values. In such cases, differences between Ct values have been estimated by the inspection of the figures. Third, these papers often include a separate analysis of the targets of amplification for those assays that include more than one target. For the most part, the different targets within a specific assay do not vary much in their Ct values, and so this level of detail will not be discussed except where necessary.

Variability Associated with Severe Acute Respiratory Syndrome Coronavirus-2 Reverse Transcription-Polymerase Chain Reaction Tests

Different RT-PCR tests for SARS-CoV-2 can yield very different Ct values. This is to be expected, given that the assays amplify different regions of the viral genome using different primers and probes and include different reagents, all of which will contribute to variations in the efficiency of the RT-PCR between assays. Reasonably comprehensive data on this issue were provided by the College of American Pathologists (CAP) Microbiology Committee in response to a paper in *Clinical Infectious Diseases*.[6] These data were collected from participants using CAP proficiency test materials. The median Ct values between different tests varied by as much as 14 cycles. Even within a single gene target on a single assay, between-laboratory results varied by up to 12 cycles. Papers in which various assays were validated or compared have similarly found differences in Ct values that ranged from 5 to slightly more than 14 cycles.[7,8] Importantly, because of high test volumes and the need for reasonable turn-around-time, many laboratories have had to run several different assays. Potentially large differences in the Ct values between assays must be considered if values are compared between assays performed in different or the same laboratory.

Variability Associated with Transport Medium and Sample Storage

The effect of dilution and storage of SARS-CoV-2 in different media, including M4, minimal essential media (MEM), phosphate-buffered saline, 0.9% saline, as well as in patient samples (sputum and bronchoalveolar lavage) has been evaluated. Briefly, 2 studies, each which included several prospective transport media or sample types, demonstrated that there was no increase greater than 2 in the Ct values for any media or sample type following storage at temperatures ranging from room temperature to −10 to −30°C during 7 days of storage.[9,10] Ct increases of slightly more than 2 were seen after storage of samples in saline after 14 days at refrigerator or freezer temperatures. In a third study, storage of SARS-CoV-2 in phosphate-buffered saline at room temperature, 4°C, −20°C, and −80°C had little effect on the Ct at 7 days.[11] From 14 to 28 days, samples with a lower level of virus (500–1000 copies/mL) had increased Ct values of slightly more than 2, and some samples became negative at room temperature, 4°C, and −20°C but not at −80°C. Samples with a higher level of virus (5000–10,000 copies/mL) did not show significant changes in the Ct values at any of these temperatures. In summary, storage at room temperature or 4C for up to a week has minimal effect on the Ct values for SARS-CoV-2, but if samples are stored longer there may be small increases of 2 to 3 Ct and lower levels of virus may become undetectable.

Variability Associated with Sample Type

There are sizable differences in the Ct values of different types of respiratory samples. Several studies compare the Ct values between different specimens of the upper respiratory tract. Saliva will be included here, because it presumably represents a mixture of saliva and mucosal upper respiratory tract secretions, with the latter presumably containing SARS-CoV-2 RNA. Because there is so much variation in the methods of sample collection and processing, the findings are generally specific to the institution whereby the study was conducted, so only a few general points can be made. First, nasopharyngeal samples usually have Ct values lower than or equal to other sample types studied. Compared with nasopharyngeal samples, nasal swabs,[12] saliva,[13,14] and oral swabs[14] have values that are approximately 5 to 7 cycles higher in some studies. Other studies have found similar Ct values for nasopharyngeal and nasal swabs,[13] or for nasopharyngeal swabs, throat swabs, sputum, and dual throat/nasopharyngeal samples.[15] A small study found that Ct values of tracheal aspirates were on average 3 cycles higher than those of nasopharyngeal swabs.[16] When the Ct values were normalized to the human RNaseP gene that was included in the assay, there was no difference between the values from tracheal aspirate and nasopharyngeal swab specimens;[16] however, the meaning of standardizing Ct values of viral RNA to human RNA is not clear.

At the time of writing, there were no studies that compared Ct values for SARS-CoV-2 PCR between samples from the upper respiratory tract and the lower respiratory tract. There are case reports and case series that show that qualitative results of bronchoalveolar lavage samples differ from those of NP swabs or other upper respiratory samples.[17] These reports usually emphasize the importance of testing lower respiratory samples to optimize the detection of SARS-CoV-2. Given these discrepant results, and the sample dilution required to collect a bronchoalveolar lavage sample, it is inevitable that there will be differences between Ct values of upper and lower respiratory samples. It is unlikely that the sample matrix will greatly affect the Ct values, at least if the method of RNA purification is adequate and consistent.[11] It is strongly recommended that the same sample type and assay be used to compare Ct values within a patient over time, unless there are sufficient local data to allow providers to make informed comparisons.

Possible Use Cases for Cycle Threshold Values for Severe Acute Respiratory Syndrome Coronavirus-2

There are 3 potential uses of Ct values that are adequately discussed in the literature to merit review. These include, first, possible use of Ct values to evaluate the progression or course of COVID-19, second, the prognostic use of Ct values as predictors of clinical severity of infection and, third, use of Ct values to determine whether a patient is potentially infectious.

Use of Cycle Threshold Values to Determine Progression of Infection

Caregivers may want to use the Ct value or multiple Ct values to determine whether the viral load is rising or falling, as a marker of whether the patient is recovering from infection. A similar, but perhaps less common use, is to use the Ct to try to determine approximately how long the patient has been infected. The utility of the Ct value for these applications depends on several things, including the average kinetics of the viral load (and associated Ct) in affected persons, the variability of these kinetics within an individual patient, and how the kinetics differ in patients who are immunocompromised. Each of these will be discussed.

A study early in the pandemic provided pooled and individual patient data on the Ct values of patients with acute COVID-19.[18] While the number of patients is small at 14, the study is valuable because the trends over time after the onset of symptoms are shown for individual patients. Nasal (mid-turbinate and nasopharyngeal) swabs or throat swabs were analyzed separately, using RT-PCR which detected regions of the N and ORF1b genes. Ct values for ORF1b were tracked over time for each patient. From this study, it is clear that aggregated Ct values are lower in the first week after symptom onset, and then higher thereafter for both specimen types, with nearly all patients having negative results by 21 days after symptom onset. However, there is marked variability in Ct values between and within patients. From the inspection of the graphs, for each of the 2 specimen types, at least 5 patients had samples that were negative followed by samples that were positive for SARS-CoV-2. Furthermore, although the aggregate Ct values rose over time, indicating falling levels of viral RNA, several patients had decreases in the Ct values of greater than 8 to 10, followed by rising Ct values or negative results. Taken together, these results indicate that results within an individual patient can be highly variable, and so using a small number of Ct values to track a patients' course may be misleading.

Numerous case reports and case series show that people who are immunocompromised can have prolonged infection with SARS-CoV-2. The largest of these includes 20 patients receiving immunosuppressive therapies for various cancers.[19] Unfortunately, the publication does not include Ct values; however, RT-PCR results are summarized and detection of replication-competent virus is presented in some detail. Viral RNA could be detected as late as 78 days after onset of symptoms (interquartile range, 24–64 days). Three of 20 patients shed replication-competent virus for more than 20 days. A smaller series, including only 3 patients with varies causes of immunosuppression and prolonged infection with SARS-CoV-2, includes Ct values.[20]

Again, as has been discussed above, there is marked variation in the Ct values over time, with apparent reductions in viral RNA being followed by increases, so that one could be misled by trying to track the course of infection by using these values. Perhaps the longest documented shedding of replication-competent SARS-CoV-2 was 238 days in an immunocompromised patient was seen in a patient with mantle cell lymphoma receiving treatment with rituximab, bendamustine, and cytarabine.[21]

Use of Cycle Threshold Values to Predict Severity of Coronavirus Disease 2019

The prognostic utility of the Ct value at or shortly after patient admission was assessed in a[22] retrospective study was performed at 2 hospitals in New York City.[22] Hospitalized patients tested positive for SARS-CoV-2 by RT-PCR using nasopharyngeal swab specimens collected within a day of admission were included. RT-PCR was performed using an assay that detects regions of the E gene and the ORF1ab gene, and Ct values from the ORF1ab gene were used to divide the patients into 3 roughly equally sized groups, with Ct values of less than 25 (high viral load), 25 to 30 (medium viral load) and greater than 30 (low viral load). Patients whose samples were positive for the E gene but negative for the ORF1ab gene were included in the low viral load group. A total of 678 patients were studied. There was a strong relationship between the viral load and in-hospital mortality, with mortality rates of 35%, 17.6%, and 6.2% for the high, medium, and low viral load groups, respectively. The proportion of patients who were intubated was similarly related to viral load, with 29.1%, 20.8%, and 14.9% for the 3 groups. Finally, multivariate analysis which included multiple risk factors such as age, race, and several comorbidities revealed a significantly increased risk of mortality in the high viral load group compared with the low viral load group, with an odds ratio of 6.05 (95% confidence interval 2.92–12.52).

Another approach has been to evaluate the prognostic value of a rising or falling Ct value over time. This was investigated in a retrospective study at a single institution.[23] Patients who presented to the Emergency Department with radiological and clinical evidence of pneumonia who had 2 or more positive SARS-CoV-2 RT-PCRs with the same assay more than 24 hours apart were included. RT-PCR was performed using an assay that amplifies the N2 and E genes, and the Ct values for the N2 results were analyzed. Clinical status was determined using the sequential organ failure assessment (SOFA) score, which includes scores for 6 organ systems and predicts clinical outcomes in critically ill patients. Only 42 patients met the inclusion criteria, which is not surprising as there was no systematic retesting required. The number of tests performed and time between tests varied, as these depended on the needs of clinical care. With these caveats, there was a relationship between the change in Ct value and the change in the SOFA score. Overall, an increase of 1 Ct value, indicating a reduction in the viral load, was associated with a decrease in the SOFA score of 0.05, indicating clinical improvement. It should be noted that many of the repeat tests were performed in patients as part of discharge planning, and this may have biased the patients studied to include those with clinical improvement. The results of this small study indicate that further research into the relationship between changes in Ct scores and changes in clinical outcomes is warranted.

A number of small studies have been conducted to evaluate the utility of the Ct value or viral load for predicting the severity of illness. The Ct value of saliva was retrospectively evaluated, using a nonstandardized clinical score, and lower Ct values were found in patients with more severe manifestations of COVID-19.[24] One study did not find a strong relationship between the Ct value and clinical outcome in 875 patients with COVID-19.[25] Patients with SARS-CoV-2 detected by RT-PCR for regions of the N1 and N2 genes were classified as having mild (no hospital admission), moderate (hospitalized in nonintensive care units) or severe (admitted to the intensive care unit) disease. The Ct values of those with moderate disease were slightly higher, on average, than those with mild or severe disease, but there was a significant overlap in the Ct distribution of the 3 groups.

Taken together, these studies indicate that patients with more severe COVID-19 tend to have lower Ct values early in the course of illness or at the time they present for medical care. However, the utility of the Ct value is limited as values overlap between groups classified by disease severity such that the values are unlikely to be useful for the care of individual patients. Furthermore, there are no data supporting the use of Ct values in making therapeutic decisions. Instead, decisions about therapy are generally guided by the clinical severity of disease.

Use of Cycle Threshold Values to Determine Infectivity

A number of studies have assessed whether lower Ct values can be used to predict who is more likely to transmit SARS-CoV-2. There have been 2 approaches to this question. Initial studies looked at the relationship between Ct values and viral culture as a proxy for infectivity. These studies required containment at BL-4 or, more recently, BL-3, and facilities for viral culture, so they could only be performed at a limited number of sites. It is important to bear in mind that the accuracy of viral culture as a surrogate for infectivity of human contacts with an index case is not known, and it is possible that viral culture overestimates or underestimates infectivity of an index case for contacts. The second, more recent approach is to link Ct values determined in routine laboratory testing to transmission events detected in epidemiologic programs meant to reduce transmission. This approach is clearly more powerful than the use of viral culture, but it also has limitations. Specifically, it cannot be definitively determined whether those contacts who become infected after exposure to an index case acquired their infection through that contact or through another contact. This could be evaluated by typing the virus, for example, with viral genome sequencing; however, such a study has not been conducted.

One of the earliest studies to evaluate the relationship between Ct values and viral culture results included 183 nasopharyngeal and sputum samples that were positive by RT-PCR for the E gene of SARS-CoV-2.[26] Samples were stored at 4°C for up to 10 hours before being processed for viral culture. Culture was performed with Vero cells, with blind subculture twice for those viral cultures not demonstrating the cytopathic effect. All samples with Ct values below 17 had growth of SARS-CoV-2 in culture, while none with Ct values greater than 34 did. No samples collected greater than 8 days after the onset of symptoms had growth of the virus in culture. A subsequent study by the same investigators expanded these data to include 3790 samples, selected and processed as above and demonstrated that samples with higher Ct values were less likely to contain SARS-CoV-2 detectable by culture.[27] However, 3% of samples with a Ct value of 35 contained detectable virus in culture. No samples with Ct values greater than 35 had positive viral cultures for SARS-CoV-2.

A separate study by Bullard and colleagues found similar results, but with some important differences. This study used 90 nasopharyngeal or endotracheal samples that were positive for SARS-CoV-2 using an RT-PCR assay targeting the E-gene.[28] The samples were in viral transport medium and they were stored at 4°C for 2 to 3 days and then frozen at −80°C for 2 to 4 weeks. Viral culture with serial dilution of the sample was performed using Vero cells. The authors showed that virus could be detected by culture as long as 8 days after the onset of symptoms and that samples positive by culture had mean Ct values of 17, compared with those that were negative by culture, which had mean Ct values of 27. All samples with virus that was detectable by culture had Ct values below 24. An excellent editorial commentary that accompanied this article pointed out that the Ct value above which no samples are positive by viral culture varies between studies, and that the effect of storing the samples on the sensitivity of viral culture is unknown.[29]

A different group evaluated the relationship between the Ct value and viral culture using 234 samples of several types, 97% of which were from the upper respiratory tract.[30] RT-PCR was performed using 5 primer-probe sets (E, RdRp, N, M, and ORF1ab) for patients in the intensive care unit and various subsets of these for other patients. Viral culture was performed using Vero cells, with terminal RT-PCR for cultures that did not show cytopathic effect. Unlike the studies discussed above, this study found a small number of samples positive in viral culture from patients with symptom onset at 17 and 18 days. For the N gene, the mean Ct value for samples with SARS-CoV-2 detectable by cytopathic effect was 25.0, while samples without cytopathic effect or terminal RT-PCR positivity had a mean Ct value of 36.9. The highest N gene Ct value for which virus could be detected in viral culture was 32. Although numerical values are not provided for the other primer-probe sets, there were much smaller differences than those for the N gene, with the exception of the ORF1ab primer-probe set. Finally, a study that used quantitative RT-PCR to measure the number of copies of viral RNA/mL found results similar to those in the studies already discussed, confirming that the Ct value is a reasonable surrogate for the burden of replication-competent virus.[31]

Taken together, these studies show that the Ct values used to predict infectivity in viral culture vary greatly, with the relevant values ranging from 24 to 35. Thus, using a specific Ct value to predict whether viral culture will be positive would have to be informed by local data. However, the culture of SARS-CoV-2 requires a biosafety level 3 laboratory according to the CDC recommendations,[32] and similar practices are recommended by the World Health Organization.[33] Many laboratories lack BSL-3 facilities, and those that have such facilities may not perform viral culture within them. Therefore, in practice, collecting such data is impractical at most institutions.

Two recent studies evaluated the relationship between Ct values for SARS-CoV-2 and transmission of infection using RT-PCR results and information from contract tracing to track transmission of infection. The smaller of the studies was conducted at Tulane University, in New Orleans, LA.[34] It included college students less than 23 years of age. Students were tested twice weekly for a 2-month period, using nasopharyngeal swab specimens that were tested within 24 hours of sample collection. The RT-PCR assay had primer-probe sets to amplify regions of the N, S, and ORF1ab genes. The Ct values for the 3 were averaged for data analysis. A total of 61,982 tests were performed on 7440 students, 602 of whom had at least one positive result. Of these, 195 were identified as index cases with one or more close contacts; 94 spread the infection to one or more close contacts and 101 did not. The surprising result was that the mean Ct value for those who spread infection was essentially the same as for those who did not (23.99 and 24.02, respectively), with very similar distributions of the Ct values. The median Ct values differed slightly, at 22.47 for those who spread infection and 24.43 for those who did not. The authors conclude that it is not practically feasible to predict who will spread infection using the Ct values as determined by the methods used.

The second study came to different conclusions, finding a strong correlation between lower Ct values in index cases and risk of transmission.[35] Data were collected from 3 high-throughput testing centers performing community testing over a 6-month period in England with linked contact tracing. The test, performed using combined nose and throat swabs, included the detection of regions of the S, N, and ORF1ab genes. Lack of amplification of the S gene was used as a surrogate for the detection of the alpha or B.1.1.7 variant of SARS-CoV-2. This large study included 1,064,004 index cases with 2,474,065 contacts, 231,498 of whom had positive RT-PCR for SARS-CoV-2. Different types of contact (household, household visitor, events/activities, work/education, and outdoors) were considered separately, and are listed in descending order of the risk of transmission. For each category of contact, there was a roughly linear relationship between the Ct value and the proportion of contacts with SARS-CoV-2 detected within 1 to 10 days following contact after the initial diagnosis of the index case. Among household contacts, for example, rates of positive SARS-CoV-2 PCR positivity were 11.7% when the index case had a Ct value of 15%, and 4.5% when the index case had a Ct value of 30. Failure of S gene amplification, indicating the likely presence of the alpha variant of SARS-CoV-2, increased the risk of transmission by 1.44- to 1.55-fold depending on the Ct value of the sample. The strengths of this study are large size and the careful analysis by contact type and SARS-CoV-2 variant, which make the results more robust than the previous study and highly generalizable. Similar results were found in a study of the risk of transmission from individuals with different viral loads (not Ct values) in respiratory samples: the secondary attack rate was 12% for index cases with 10^6 or fewer copies of RNA per mL, but 24% for index cases with 10^{10} or greater.[36]

Recommendations on Reporting Cycle Threshold Values

The decisions of whether and when to report Ct values should be made by the laboratory directors in consultation with local experts in compliance and departmental leadership. If the leadership group decides that Ct values should be reported, several other decisions should be made before proceeding. The first task is to decide whether all results will be reported or if they will be selectively reported, that is, on request. Reporting of all results may cause confusion among caregivers who do not know how to interpret the information; therefore, selective reporting would seem to be the better choice. Second, if reporting is to be conducted selectively, it must be determined who may request the information. One option would be to work with the infectious diseases practitioners at the institution and provide them with the information needed to understand and use these results. If caregivers from other specialties request Ct values, they could be directed to involve infectious diseases specialists so that the information is used appropriately. The third task involves providing the supporting information necessary to help providers correctly interpret a Ct value. Basic information to be provided includes the fact that lower Ct values indicate higher concentrations of viral RNA and that a difference of 3 Ct values indicates approximately a 10-fold different level of viral RNA. Local data about RT-PCR efficiency might be used to provide a more precise relationship between these values. An understanding of the factors underlying the variability of Ct values is essential, so that simple mistakes, such as comparing Ct values from different specimen types, are avoided. Finally, basic statistical values of the Ct values obtained in the laboratory should be used to understand the Ct value. These could include, for example, the mean, median and interquartile ranges for symptomatic patients' results.

CLINICS CARE POINTS

- Because there are several sources of variability in the Ct values for SARS-CoV-2, clinical staff should work closely with laboratory staff to interpret Ct values for individual patients.

- The sources of variability in Ct values for SARS-CoV-2 vary in the size of variability that they introduce. The greatest potential for variability in the Ct values is comparison of Ct values from different assays. Variability of Ct values can be mitigated by comparing values only when they are from the same assay, and by taking steps to ensure that samples tested are of the same kind and are stored in a manner that will preserve the viral RNA.
- Potential applications of Ct values for SARS-CoV-2 in patients include evaluation of the course of the infection, prognosis of the infection and assessment of infectivity.

DISCLOSURE

The author has nothing to disclose.

REFERENCES

1. Center for systems Science and Engineering (CSSE) at Johns Hopkins University (JHU). COVID-19 Dashboard. Available at: https://coronavirus.jhu.edu/map.html. Accessed February 2, 2022.
2. Important issues to consider before interpreting and Applying Ct values in clinical practice. 2021. Available at: https://www.amp.org/about/news-room/amp-blog-content/important-issues-to-consider-before-interpreting-and-applying-ct-values-in-clinical-practice/. Accessed July 14, 2021.
3. Values Ct. What they are and how they can be used. 2021. Available at: https://www.aphl.org/programs/preparedness/Crisis-Management/Documents/APHL-COVID19-Ct-Values.pdf. Accessed July 14, 2021.
4. AACC recommendation for reporting SARS-CoV-2 cycle threshold (CT) values. 2021. Available at: https://www.aacc.org/science-and-research/covid-19-resources/statements-on-covid-19-testing/aacc-recommendation-for-reporting-sars-cov-2-cycle-threshold-ct-values. Accessed July 14, 2021.
5. Mandatory reporting of COVID-19 laboratory test results: reporting of cycle threshold values. Available at: https://www.flhealthsource.gov/files/Laboratory-Reporting-CT-Values-12032020.pdf. Accessed July 14, 2021.
6. Rhoads D, Peaper DR, She RC, et al. College of American Pathologists (CAP) Microbiology Committee Perspective: Caution must Be used in interpreting the cycle threshold (Ct) value. Clin Infect Dis 2021;72(10):e685–6.
7. Hirschhorn JW, Kegl A, Dickerson T, et al. Verification and validation of SARS-CoV-2 assay performance on the Abbott m2000 and Alinity m systems. J Clin Microbiol 2021;(5):59. https://doi.org/10.1128/jcm.03119-20.
8. Perchetti GA, Pepper G, Shrestha L, et al. Performance characteristics of the Abbott Alinity m SARS-CoV-2 assay. J Clin Virol Jul 2021;140:104869. https://doi.org/10.1016/j.jcv.2021.104869.
9. Rodino KG, Espy MJ, Buckwalter SP, et al. Evaluation of saline, phosphate-buffered saline, and Minimum essential medium as potential Alternatives to viral transport media for SARS-CoV-2 testing. J Clin Microbiol 2020;(6):58. https://doi.org/10.1128/jcm.00590-20.
10. Rogers AA, Baumann RE, Borillo GA, et al. Evaluation of transport media and specimen transport Conditions for the detection of SARS-CoV-2 by Use of Real-time reverse transcription-PCR. J Clin Microbiol 2020;(8):58. https://doi.org/10.1128/jcm.00708-20.
11. Perchetti GA, Nalla AK, Huang ML, et al. Validation of SARS-CoV-2 detection across multiple specimen types. J Clin Virol 2020;128:104438. https://doi.org/10.1016/j.jcv.2020.104438.

12. Callahan C, Lee RA, Lee GR, et al. Nasal swab performance by collection timing, Procedure, and method of transport for patients with SARS-CoV-2. J Clin Microbiol 2021. https://doi.org/10.1128/jcm.00569-21. Jcm0056921.

13. Griesemer SB, Van Slyke G, Ehrbar D, et al. Evaluation of specimen types and saliva Stabilization Solutions for SARS-CoV-2 testing. J Clin Microbiol 2021;(5): 59. https://doi.org/10.1128/jcm.01418-20.

14. Plantamura J, Bousquet A, Otto MP, et al. Performances, feasibility and acceptability of nasopharyngeal swab, saliva and oral-self sampling swab for the detection of severe acute respiratory syndrome coronavirus 2. Eur J Clin Microbiol Infect Dis 2021;1–8. https://doi.org/10.1007/s10096-021-04269-4.

15. Sharma K, Aggarwala P, Gandhi D, et al. Comparative analysis of various clinical specimens in detection of SARS-CoV-2 using rRT-PCR in new and follow up cases of COVID-19 infection: Quest for the best choice. PLoS One 2021;16(4): e0249408. https://doi.org/10.1371/journal.pone.0249408.

16. Miranda RL, Guterres A, de Azeredo Lima CH, et al. Misinterpretation of viral load in COVID-19 clinical outcomes. Virus Res 2021;296:198340. https://doi.org/10. 1016/j.virusres.2021.198340.

17. Baron A, Hachem M, Tran Van Nhieu J, et al. Bronchoalveolar lavage in patients with COVID-19 with Invasive Mechanical Ventilation for acute respiratory distress syndrome. Ann Am Thorac Soc 2021;18(4):723–6.

18. Zou L, Ruan F, Huang M, et al. SARS-CoV-2 viral load in upper respiratory specimens of infected patients. N Engl J Med 2020;382(12):1177–9.

19. Aydillo T, Gonzalez-Reiche AS, Aslam S, et al. Shedding of viable SARS-CoV-2 after immunosuppressive therapy for cancer. N Engl J Med 2020;383(26):2586–8.

20. Tarhini H, Recoing A, Bridier-Nahmias A, et al. Long-term severe acute respiratory syndrome coronavirus 2 (SARS-CoV-2) Infectiousness among three immunocompromised patients: from prolonged viral shedding to SARS-CoV-2 Superinfection. J Infect Dis 2021;223(9):1522–7.

21. Taramasso L, Sepulcri C, Mikulska M, et al. Duration of isolation and precautions in immunocompromised patients with COVID-19. J Hosp Infect 2021;111:202–4.

22. Magleby R, Westblade LF, Trzebucki A, et al. Impact of SARS-CoV-2 viral load on risk of intubation and mortality among hospitalized patients with coronavirus disease 2019. Clin Infect Dis 2020. https://doi.org/10.1093/cid/ciaa851.

23. Zacharioudakis IM, Zervou FN, Prasad PJ, et al. Association of SARS-CoV-2 genomic load trends with clinical status in COVID-19: a retrospective analysis from an academic hospital center in New York City. PLoS One 2020;15(11): e0242399. https://doi.org/10.1371/journal.pone.0242399.

24. Aydin S, Benk IG, Geckil AA. May viral load detected in saliva in the early stages of infection be a prognostic indicator in COVID-19 patients? J Virol Methods 2021;294:114198. https://doi.org/10.1016/j.jviromet.2021.114198.

25. Faíco-Filho KS, Passarelli VC, Bellei N. Is higher viral load in SARS-CoV-2 associated with death? Am J Trop Med Hyg 2020;103(5):2019–21.

26. La Scola B, Le Bideau M, Andreani J, et al. Viral RNA load as determined by cell culture as a management tool for discharge of SARS-CoV-2 patients from infectious disease wards. Eur J Clin Microbiol Infect Dis 2020;39(6):1059–61.

27. Jaafar R, Aherfi S, Wurtz N, et al. Correlation between 3790 quantitative polymerase chain reaction-Positives samples and positive cell cultures, including 1941 severe acute respiratory syndrome coronavirus 2 Isolates. Clin Infect Dis 2021; 72(11):e921. https://doi.org/10.1093/cid/ciaa1491.

28. Bullard J, Dust K, Funk D, et al. Predicting infectious severe acute respiratory syndrome coronavirus 2 from diagnostic samples. Clin Infect Dis 2020;71(10): 2663–6.

29. Binnicker MJ. Can the severe acute respiratory syndrome coronavirus 2 polymerase chain reaction cycle threshold value and time from symptom onset to testing predict infectivity? Clin Infect Dis 2020;71(10):2667–8.

30. Basile K, McPhie K, Carter I, et al. Cell-based culture of SARS-CoV-2 informs infectivity and safe de-isolation assessments during COVID-19. Clin Infect Dis 2020. https://doi.org/10.1093/cid/ciaa1579.

31. van Kampen JJA, van de Vijver D, Fraaij PLA, et al. Duration and key determinants of infectious virus shedding in hospitalized patients with coronavirus disease-2019 (COVID-19). Nat Commun 2021;12(1):267. https://doi.org/10. 1038/s41467-020-20568-4.

32. Biosafety for specimen Handling. Available at: https://www.cdc.gov/coronavirus/ 2019-ncov/lab/lab-biosafety-guidelines.html. Accessed July 14, 2021.

33. Laboratory biosafety guidance related to coronavirus disease (COVID-19): Interim guidance. 2021. Available at: https://www.who.int/publications/i/item/ WHO-WPE-GIH-2021.1. Accessed July 14, 2021.

34. Tian D, Lin Z, Kriner EM, et al. Ct values do not predict SARS-CoV-2 Transmissibility in college students. J Mol Diagn 2021. https://doi.org/10.1016/j.jmoldx. 2021.05.012.

35. Lee LYW, Rozmanowski S, Pang M, et al. SARS-CoV-2 infectivity by viral load, S gene variants and demographic factors and the utility of lateral flow devices to prevent transmission. Clin Infect Dis 2021. https://doi.org/10.1093/cid/ciab421.

36. Marks M, Millat-Martinez P, Ouchi D, et al. Transmission of COVID-19 in 282 clusters in Catalonia, Spain: a cohort study. Lancet Infect Dis 2021;21(5):629–36.

Performance of Non-nasopharyngeal Sample Types for Molecular Detection of SARS-CoV-2

Benjamin Kukull, MD[a], Salika M. Shakir, PhD[a,b],
Kimberly E. Hanson, MD, MHS[b,c],*

KEYWORDS

- SARS-CoV-2 • COVID-19 • Molecular diagnostic • Nasopharyngeal swab
- Non-NP respiratory specimen • Alternative specimen

KEY POINTS

- Although SARS-CoV-2 RNA can be detected in a variety of different body fluids, infectious virus particles are rarely recovered outside of the respiratory tract.
- The sensitivity of SARS-CoV-2 detection in non-nasopharyngeal samples varies with regards to the timeline of infection, disease severity, body site, and specimen collection method.
- Anterior nasal swabs, midturbinate swabs, combined nasal and oropharyngeal swabs, or saliva are acceptable alternatives to nasopharyngeal swabs for SARS-CoV-2 diagnosis and screening.
- The frequent shedding of viral RNA in stool provides rationale for using wastewater in public health surveillance. In contrast, SARS-CoV-2 is rarely detectable in blood and asymptomatic blood donors do not currently require screening.

INTRODUCTION

COVID-19 is predominantly a respiratory disease characterized by a dysregulated inflammatory response to a viral infection with presentations ranging from asymptomatic to multiorgan failure and death. The tropism of SARS-CoV-2, the virus that causes COVID-19, for various tissues is conferred by the widely expressed surface proteins, angiotensin-converting enzyme 2 (ACE2) and transmembrane serine protease 2 (TMPRSS2), which function as the receptor and coreceptor for cell entry,

[a] Department of Pathology, Cascade Pathology Services/Legacy Health, Portland, OR, USA;
[b] ARUP Laboratories, Salt Lake City, UT, USA; [c] Department of Medicine, Division of Infectious Diseases, University of Utah School of Medicine, Salt Lake City, UT, USA
* Corresponding author. University of Utah, School of Medicine, 30 N 1900 E, Salt Lake City, UT 84132, USA
E-mail address: kim.hanson@hsc.utah.edu

Clin Lab Med 42 (2022) 249–259
https://doi.org/10.1016/j.cll.2022.02.002
0272-2712/22/© 2022 Elsevier Inc. All rights reserved.

labmed.theclinics.com

respectively. ACE2 is present on various cells of the respiratory tract, gastrointestinal (GI) tract, vasculature, and on epithelial cells of various other organs.[1] Owing to the potential for multiorgan system involvement and concerns for viral transmissibility, many studies have looked for detectable SARS-CoV-2 RNA in a variety of different body sites. Here, we review the findings and clinical utility of SARS-CoV-2 nucleic acid detection in commonly tested non-nasopharyngeal (NP) specimens.

RESPIRATORY TRACT SPECIMENS
Performance Characteristics of Non-nasopharyngeal Upper Respiratory Specimens

Nasopharyngeal swab (NPS) collection was initially assumed to be the preferred specimen type for SARS-CoV-2 detection. However, NPS collection is relatively invasive, requires trained health care workers wearing personal protective equipment (PPE), and is subject to sampling error. In addition, dedicated NPSs were in short supply during the pandemic. Consequently, alternative, non-NP upper respiratory tract (URT) sampling approaches including use of anterior nares (AN) swabs, midturbinate (MT) swabs, oropharyngeal (OP) swabs, and saliva were explored to mitigate one or more of the challenges associated with NPS collection (**Table 1**).

Saliva

Saliva was noted to be a promising specimen type early in the pandemic because SARS-CoV-2 was shown to be reproducibly detectable in the oral secretions of infected individuals, it is a noninvasive sample type that requires minimal supervision to obtain, and collection potentially minimizes health care personnel exposure to

Table 1
Recommendations of appropriate sample types for SARS-CoV-2 viral RNA testing

Sample Type	Diagnosis	Screening	Public Health Surveillance[a]	Not Clinically Useful
NP	×	×	×	
Saliva	×	×	×	
OP	×	×	×	
AN	×	×	×	
AN/MT	×	×	×	
Sputum	×			
ETS	×			
BAL	×			
Stool			× (Wastewater)	
Blood				×
CSF				×
Urine				×
Other blood fluids[b]				×

Abbreviations: BAL, bronchoalveolar lavage; CSF, cerebrospinal fluid; ETS, endotracheal secretions.
   [a] Public health surveillance refers to testing of specimens that have no patient identification, are not reported to health care providers, and can therefore take place in non–CLIA-certified laboratories. The CDC and US Department of Health and Human Services oversees a collaborative effort for testing untreated wastewater and primary sludge in selected communities. Another example of public health surveillance includes genomic screening for novel viral variants.
   [b] Includes reported studies of amniotic fluid, breast milk, conjunctival secretions, semen, and vaginal secretions.

infectious aerosols. In addition, saliva reduces the need for swabs and transport media. However, saliva is a complex matrix that can be difficult to work within the clinical laboratory. Automated sample-to-result platforms designed for swab collection tubes may not be amenable to use with saliva samples and saliva may require heat or chemical inactivation before testing.[2]

Overall test performance

Viral load is generally highest in saliva within the first week of infection.[3–5] Notably, SARS-CoV-2 RNA can be detected in saliva earlier and for a longer duration of time than NPS.[4] Multiple meta-analyses have compared SARS-CoV-2 RNA detection rates in saliva to NPS as well as assessed the impact of different saliva collection methods on test performance. Positivity rates across 4528 paired saliva and NPS samples were similar (88% [95% confidence interval (CI), 81%-93%] vs 94% [95% CI, 90%-98%] for saliva vs NPS, respectively).[2] Another meta-analysis showed similar nucleic acid amplification test (NAAT) pooled sensitivity for saliva versus NPS (sensitivity 83.2% [95% CI, 74.7%–91.4%] vs 84.8% [95% CI, 76.8%-92.4%]) and specificity (99.2% [95% CI, 95.2%–99.8%] vs 98.9% [95% CI, 97.4%-99.8%]), respectively.[6] Of note, saliva performed better than NPS in some studies highlighting the limitation of NPS as the gold standard.[5,7,8] Test characteristics varied substantially across different studies comparing saliva to NPS likely as a result of variability in the timing of testing relative to infection onset, severity of illness, and efficiency of nucleic acid extraction and amplification.

Collection method

Several different saliva collection methods have been assessed including passive drool/spit, coughed or deep-throat saliva, oral rinses, and fluid from oral cavity swabs. Saliva tests authorized by the Food and Drug Administration (FDA) for emergency use require collection tubes with stabilization or inactivation buffers. However, several studies have demonstrated high SARS-CoV-2 RNA stability in saliva collected in tubes without these additives, which may simplify specimen collection and reduce cost.[9,10]

Drool and spit methods. Recent meta-analyses reported that drool or spit protocols had an overall positive detection rate of 86% (95% CI, 78%–92%) compared with 95% for NPS (95% CI, 93%–97%) and was superior to oral fluid collected by swabs from the gumline.[2]

Saliva with coughing. Studies comparing coughed or deep-throat saliva had a positive detection rate of 94% compared with NPS, suggesting that these specimens may contain more virus than drool/spit saliva.[11,12] However, forced cough requires use of PPE to protect health care workers against potential infectious aerosols. Saliva that is excessively mucoid may lead to increased pipetting errors on automated systems necessitating a dilution or pretreatment/chemical digestion of the samples. Studies have shown comparable positivity and stability between undiluted or diluted saliva samples.[2]

Oral rinses. Few studies have evaluated oral rinses or gargles for SARS-CoV-2 detection. Saline gargles were suggested for hospitalized patients who were unable to produce sputum and for those patients who were unable to produce sufficient amounts of saliva.[13] Saline gargles appear to have comparable sensitivity to NPS collections for symptomatic patients.[14,15] In one study, the sensitivity and specificity of saline gargle were observed to be more than 90% and 98%, respectively, compared with NPS.[14] In contrast, another study reported a reduced sensitivity (63%) for oral rinses versus undiluted saliva (94.1%) relative to NPS. These studies differed in collection and testing methods. Oral rinses or gargles may be easier to collect than other forms of saliva, but additional data are required before this approach can be recommended.

Host factors

Host factors have also been shown to impact SARS CoV-2 test performance.

Symptomatic versus asymptomatic individuals. Symptomatic and asymptomatic individuals infected with SARS-CoV-2 are thought to harbor similar amounts of virus. However, paired comparisons of saliva to NPS for the detection of SARS-CoV-2 RNA in symptomatic and asymptomatic individuals have produced incongruent results potentially as a result of the timing of testing relative to symptom onset. One meta-analysis demonstrated high and comparable sensitivities of saliva in symptomatic and asymptomatic individuals (88% vs 87%, respectively), whereas NPS demonstrated higher sensitivity in symptomatic (96%) versus asymptomatic populations (73%).[2]

Pediatric patients. Relatively few saliva studies have been performed in the pediatric population and these reports differ widely in terms of sample size, collection, and testing methods.[2,16] The most robust studies, however, demonstrate comparable sensitivities between saliva and NPS in children (∼82% vs 87%, respectively).[17,18] Overall, the subset of pediatric studies suggests that both NPS and saliva are acceptable sample types.

Nasal Swabs

Nasal swabs, when swabs are available, are also an attractive alternative to NPS because they are less invasive and can be collected by the patient. Nasal specimens are approved for use with many commercially available NAATs, but there are conflicting data on their test performance compared with NPS. Nasal swab specimens (including AN and MT) are generally obtained from both nares. The CDC's interim guidelines for COVID-19 clinical specimens[19] differentiate between AN and MT collection by the distance of swab insertion into the nostril, but these terms are often used interchangeably in studies comparing their performance to NPS.

A recent meta-analysis showed that nasal swabs (either AN or MT) had a lower positive detection rate of 82% (95% CI, 73%–90%) compared with 98% (95% CI, 96%–100%) for NPS, and there was modest agreement (79%) between the 2 specimen types. Detection with nasal swabs was highest in individuals with symptoms ≤ 7 days (88% [95% CI, 74%–95%]).[2]

As observed with saliva collection, substantial heterogeneity was observed in studies comparing nasal and NPS test performance. In addition to the timing of testing, swab type has also been shown to affect test sensitivity. Specifically, foam or flocked nasal swabs performed better than unflocked or polyester swab specimens (percent positivity 90%, [95% CI, 81%–97%] versus 77% [95% CI, 55%–93%], respectively),[20,21] whereas the person collecting the sample (self vs health care worker) and use of transport media (dry swab vs diluted) do not appear to impact detection rates.[20,21,2]

Oropharyngeal and Dual Anterior Nares/Oropharyngeal Swabs

A meta-analysis of OP swab and NPS samples in symptomatic patients found similar positivity rates (84% [95% CI, 57%–100%] vs 88% [95% CI, 73%–98%], respectively), but the overall agreement between the 2 sample types was only 68% (95% CI, 36%–93%).[2] Two additional meta-analyses showed that combining both OP and AN swabs in a single collection tube improves the rate of SARS-CoV-2 detection by molecular methods (sensitivity 97% and specificity 99%).[2,22] In addition, supervised self-collected OP/AN swabs had comparable sensitivity to Health care worker (HCW)-collected OP/AN swabs using 3 different molecular testing platforms.[23]

Performance Characteristics of Lower Respiratory Tract Specimens

The lower respiratory tract (LRT) is considered to be the most sensitive anatomic site for SARS-CoV-2 RNA detection,[24] possibly due to reports suggesting that higher levels of RNA are present in this anatomic compartment.[25,26] However, this observation may be biased by severe presentations, which presumably are associated with higher virion burden, were more likely to have LRT testing performed. Viral RNA loads and infectious particles peak in the first week of infection in the LRT (**Fig. 1**),[27–29] but the shedding of viral RNA and infectious virus particles can be prolonged in this compartment.[25,28] Prolonged shedding is thought to be more pronounced in severe disease and in the immunocompromised. These patients may yield positive test results for several months beyond the resolution of symptoms,[25,26,30] and the clinical and infection control significance of this is not fully known. Additional limitations of LRT testing include the need for clinical laboratories to validate additional sample

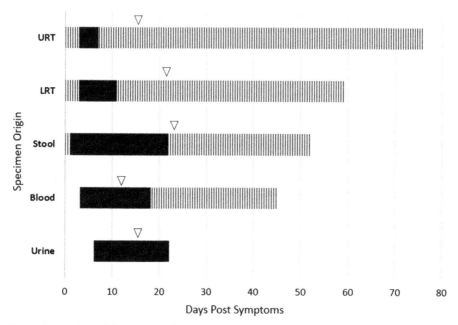

Fig. 1. Illustration of the estimated reported ranges of detection of SARS-CoV-2 RNA in specimens from different anatomic regions in symptomatic patients. Ranges of detection are approximations according to several meta-analyses of SARS-CoV-2 detection by RT-PCR.[25–27,29] This datum has not been standardized between studies. The peak Ct range (*black area*), average duration of detection (*arrowhead*), and total reported detectable range (*black + vertical line areas*) of SARS-CoV-2 RNA are averages of published data from the same references and were inferred in these cases from studies with serial RT-PCR testing and reported Ct values for these specimen types. Upper and lower respiratory tract specimens peak most often in the first week, whereas the peak range for non-respiratory specimens is not well-defined. Note that detection of viral RNA in blood and urine is infrequent, and average and extreme ranges overlap. Specific specimen types were omitted due to a relative lack of quality, high power data for meaningful comparisons.

types that may not be covered under emergency use authorizations for commercially available SARS-CoV-2 NAATs. Common LRT sampling strategies are also associated with risk for aerosol generation and some (eg, bronchoscopy) are invasive.

Few studies have directly compared the diagnostic yield of various LRT specimen types to one another or to NPS collected from the same patient at the time. In one study of greater than 1000 patients where exposure history, symptoms, and radiology were used as a reference method to confirm COVID-19, the highest viral RNA detection rates were in bronchoalveolar lavage (BAL) specimens (93%), followed by sputum (72%) and then nasal swabs (63%).[31]

Sputum

Sputum can be collected during voluntary expectoration or by induction. However, COVID-19 patients may not have a productive cough, and sputum induction has generally been avoided because of the risk of generating infectious aerosols. Thick mucus might also add to the difficulty in isolating nucleic acids in some specimens. Classic nucleic acid isolation techniques in sputum have included treatments with reducing agents and mucolytic enzymes to reduce viscosity and increase nucleic acid yield. Manufacturer-approved sterile collection tubes should also be used for molecular testing, as certain synthetic polymers can bind nucleic acid and interfere with the yield of extraction.

Endotracheal Aspiration

Endotracheal aspiration (ETA) specimens can be acquired from intubated patients or through a tracheostomy tube. To collect this specimen type, a catheter is placed through the endotracheal tube, and secretions are usually aspirated into a sterile pre-attached specimen trap. ETAs are sometimes collected when more invasive testing strategies are not possible and may be less likely to produce aerosols compared with bronchoscopy. ETA samples are thought to have similar sensitivities compared to sputum, but relatively little performance data for ETA exist.[31,32]

Bronchoalveolar Lavage and Bronchial Washings

BAL sampling is performed during minimally flexible bronchoscopy by instilling a specific amount of saline and aspirating this volume for testing.[33] For example, a lavage volume of 100 mL samples approximately 1.5% to 3.0% of the lung, or approximately one million alveoli. BAL may be performed with or without established intubation and many centers tried to avoid these procedures because of aerosol generation. However, reports of increased SARS-CoV-2 detection sensitivity of this specimen type provide diagnostic rationale, especially in the case of pneumonia with negative URT testing and high radiologic and/or clinical suspicion of COVID-19.[34] BAL sampling has been shown to have the highest rate of detection compared with all other samples in systematic comparison studies as well as in late clinical detection and persistent disease.[26,31] BAL testing may also be particularly useful when coinfections need to be ruled out with high confidence.

Summary of Current COVID-19 Diagnostic Guidelines for Respiratory Specimens

Owing to convenience, URT testing is preferred as the first-line test. However, LRT testing may also be useful, especially when URT testing is negative but a high clinical suspicion for COVID-19 pneumonia remains. Current IDSA guidelines recommend collection of NPS, MTS, ANS, saliva, or a combined AN/OP swabs rather than OP swab alone as a first test for all symptomatic persons.[35]

NONRESPIRATORY SPECIMENS
Stool

Following the respiratory tract, the GI system is the next most affected organ system by COVID-19, which is believed to be related to the viral tropism of various cell types in the GI tract.[1] Several studies estimate that GI symptoms in COVID-19 patients may be present in approximately 10% to 50% of patients.[36,37] The presentation of GI symptoms ranges from asymptomatic to severe disturbances, which in some cases is reported independent of the severity of the respiratory disease.[28] SARS-CoV-2 RNA has been detected from various GI specimens including gastric lavage stool, and anorectal swabs, but stool is the most reported specimen type. Certainly, collection and reverse transcription–polymerase chain reaction (PCR) needs to be carefully standardized to ensure meaningful data in this highly variable sample type. There are many natural constituents of stool that degrade viral RNA and inhibit PCR reactions, including degradative enzymes, bile salts, and dietary polysaccharides.

Despite the natural challenges with this specimen type, viral RNA has been detected in stool over a broad timeframe regardless of GI symptoms or disease severity.[25,26] The detection of viral RNA in stool does not seem to correlate with respiratory viral RNA detection or vice versa.[25,28,38] There is significant heterogeneity between studies and meta-analyses with regards to clinical sensitivity (approximate range, 30%–60%) and detection timeframes (see **Fig. 1**).[25,26,37,38] In one meta-analysis, there was reported viral shedding in several studies at least 4 weeks after symptom onset.[25] Patients without GI symptoms may still have detectable viral RNA in a stool sample much beyond the resolution of COVID-19 symptoms.[26,29,36] A minority of specimens with detectable viral RNA in stool also has yielded infectious virus in culture, suggesting that fecal-oral transmission of COVID-19 may be theoretically possible even though most of these specimens are considered noninfectious.[31,38] Owing to the relatively high abundance of viral RNA shedding in stool samples, several population studies have also shown that wastewater and sewage may serve as a useful sample for population screening, which has been used in several public health surveillance strategies.[39] This approach to a massively "pooled" specimen may be useful for predicting outbreaks on the population level.

Blood

As with stool, meta-analyses of the detection of SARS-CoV-2 RNA in serum or plasma have significant heterogeneity and this specimen type is not recommended for diagnostic testing.[19,40] When compared with all respiratory sample types, the clinical sensitivity of blood specimens for COVID-19 infection is consistently much lower (~0%-45%), and positive detection appears to correlate with disease severity and mortality in a few reports.[26,29,41] When testing blood, molecular tests should exclude samples with residual, well-described, and ubiquitous PCR inhibitors from their protocols, such as heme and heparin.

Viral RNA detection surprisingly has been detected up to 60 days in serum,[25] but most studies report an average detection timeframe of 3 to 18 days (see **Fig. 1**).[26] Despite the potential prolonged detection of viral RNA in these specimen types, no live virus has been successfully isolated from serum in these reports.[26,28] Recently, a massive study of 258,000 blood donations showed very infrequent detection of SARS-CoV-2 RNA (1.16/100,000), and no infectivity was demonstrated in cell culture.[42] Considering an extremely low risk of COVID-19 transmission from blood, FDA does not currently require screening routine asymptomatic blood donors for SARS-CoV-2 or after 14 days of resolution of COVID-19 symptoms.[43]

Other Body Fluids

SARS-CoV-2 testing has been performed on the body fluids that are discussed in **Table 1**, but data currently exist as case reports without paired comparisons to a reference method or standardized molecular detection methods. None of the fluids discussed in **Table 1** are currently considered clinically useful for the detection of SARS-CoV-2.

Cerebrospinal fluid (CSF) testing has been reported in several studies and analyzed in meta-analyses, with rare reports detected viral RNA.[26] It is not clear if these instances represent a true positive, viremia with CSF blood contamination, or breach of the blood-brain barrier due to systemic inflammation, or other vascular pathology. There appears to be no clinical indication for CSF sampling in COVID-19 patients, yet some laboratories may still offer this testing as a validated specimen type. There is a similar scenario with urine, where little to no detection has been reported.[44,45] Detected viral RNA could represent primary renal involvement or viremia with widespread vascular pathology. Of note, ACE2 and TMPRSS2 are coexpressed in renal tubules and podocytes,[46] and primary COVID-19–associated kidney pathology has been proposed.[47] There is also inconclusive or conflicting evidence for the true involvement of SARS-CoV-2 in amniotic fluid, breast milk, conjunctival secretions, semen, and vaginal secretions.[26]

SUMMARY

SARS-CoV-2 viral RNA shedding is temporally dynamic and differs between respiratory and distant anatomic sites. Standardized collection processes and appropriate testing rationale are essential, regardless of specimen type. The vast majority of test performance data come from assessments of various URT specimen types. URT samples are easy to obtain and accurate in comparison with NP testing, but it should be noted that NP testing is an imperfect gold standard and there may be circumstances where alternatives are preferred. There is also clear utility in testing the LRT, especially when URT testing is negative and there is high clinical suspicion for COVID-19 pneumonia. Stool testing is not as clinically sensitive in COVID-19 patients as respiratory specimens, but studies of sewage show continual promise as a population-level screening tool. The presence of SARS-CoV-2 viral RNA in blood and other body fluids appears to be transient in the most severely ill patients, shows great variability, and should not be performed to track disease progression. A shared knowledge of the limitations of molecular tests is also clinically essential as we face a landscape of novel variants with unpredictable testing parameters. Constant adaptation to these viral dynamics will be required in addition to higher quality data for emerging detection technologies.

CLINICS CARE POINTS

- Non-nasopharyngeal upper respiratory tract specimens such as nasal swab or saliva may be used for molecular detection of SARS-CoV-2.

- Various factors including timing of onset of symptoms, host factors, and method of collection may affect test sensitivity for non-nasopharyngeal specimens.

- Lower respiratory tract specimens like BAL are a useful diagnostic specimen in patients with COVID-19 pneumonia.-Testing of stool and other non-respiratory specimens has a limited role in the diagnosis of COVID-19.

- Testing of stool and other non-respiratory specimens has a limited role in the diagnosis of COVID-19.
- Further studies are needed to understand the effect of SARS-CoV-2 variants on the detection rate of non-nasopharyngeal specimens.

DISCLOSURE

The authors have nothing to disclose.

REFERENCES

1. Salamanna F, Maglio M, Landini MP, et al. Body Localization of ACE-2: on the Trail of the Keyhole of SARS-CoV-2. Front Med 2020;7:594495.
2. Lee RA, Herigon JC, Benedetti A, et al. Performance of saliva, oropharyngeal swabs, and nasal swabs for SARS-CoV-2 molecular detection: a systematic review and meta-analysis. J Clin Microbiol 2021;59(5).
3. Teo AKJ, Choudhury Y, Tan IB, et al. Saliva is more sensitive than nasopharyngeal or nasal swabs for diagnosis of asymptomatic and mild COVID-19 infection. Sci Rep 2021;11(1):3134.
4. Williams E, Bond K, Zhang B, et al. Saliva as a Noninvasive specimen for detection of SARS-CoV-2. J Clin Microbiol 2020;58(8).
5. Wyllie AL, Fournier J, Casanovas-Massana A, et al. Saliva or nasopharyngeal swab specimens for detection of SARS-CoV-2. N Engl J Med 2020;383(13): 1283–6.
6. Butler-Laporte G, Lawandi A, Schiller I, et al. Comparison of saliva and nasopharyngeal swab nucleic acid amplification testing for detection of SARS-CoV-2: a systematic review and meta-analysis. JAMA Intern Med 2021;181(3):353–60.
7. Hanson KE, Barker AP, Hillyard DR, et al. Self-collected anterior nasal and saliva specimens versus healthcare worker-collected nasopharyngeal swabs for the molecular detection of SARS-CoV-2. J Clin Microbiol 2020;58(11).
8. Kojima N, Turner F, Slepnev V, et al. Self-collected oral fluid and nasal swab specimens demonstrate comparable sensitivity to Clinician-collected nasopharyngeal swab specimens for the detection of SARS-CoV-2. Clin Infect Dis 2021;73(9).
9. Griesemer SB, Van Slyke G, Ehrbar D, et al. Evaluation of specimen types and saliva stabilization Solutions for SARS-CoV-2 testing. J Clin Microbiol 2021;59(5).
10. Ott IM, Strine MS, Watkins AE, et al. Stability of SARS-CoV-2 RNA in Nonsupplemented saliva. Emerg Infect Dis 2021;27(4):1146–50.
11. Procop GW, Shrestha NK, Vogel S, et al. A Direct comparison of Enhanced saliva to nasopharyngeal swab for the detection of SARS-CoV-2 in symptomatic patients. J Clin Microbiol 2020;58(11).
12. Rao M, Rashid FA, Sabri F, et al. Comparing nasopharyngeal swab and early Morning saliva for the identification of severe acute respiratory Syndrome coronavirus 2 (SARS-CoV-2). Clin Infect Dis 2021;72(9):e352–6.
13. Saito M, Adachi E, Yamayoshi S, et al. Gargle lavage as a Safe and sensitive alternative to swab samples to Diagnose COVID-19: a case report in Japan. Clin Infect Dis 2020;71(15):893–4.
14. Goldfarb DM, Tilley P, Al-Rawahi GN, et al. Self-collected saline gargle samples as an alternative to health care worker-collected nasopharyngeal swabs for COVID-19 diagnosis in outpatients. J Clin Microbiol 2021;59(4).

15. Kandel CE, Young M, Serbanescu MA, et al. Detection of severe acute respiratory coronavirus virus 2 (SARS-CoV-2) in outpatients: a multicenter comparison of self-collected saline gargle, oral swab, and combined oral-anterior nasal swab to a provider collected nasopharyngeal swab. Infect Control Hosp Epidemiol 2021;1–5.

16. Chong CY, Kam KQ, Li J, et al. Saliva is not a useful diagnostic specimen in children with Coronavirus Disease 2019. Clin Infect Dis 2021;73(9).

17. Al Suwaidi H, Senok A, Varghese R, et al. Saliva for molecular detection of SARS-CoV-2 in school-age children. Clin Microbiol Infect 2021;27(9):1330–5.

18. Yee R, Truong TT, Pannaraj PS, et al. Saliva is a promising alternative specimen for the detection of SARS-CoV-2 in children and Adults. J Clin Microbiol 2021;59(2).

19. Interim CDC. Guidelines for collecting, Handling, and testing clinical specimens for COVID-19. 2020. Available at: https://www.cdc.gov/coronavirus/2019-ncov/lab/guidelines-clinical-specimens.html. Accessed April 22nd, 2021.

20. Tu YP, Jennings R, Hart B, et al. Swabs collected by patients or health care workers for SARS-CoV-2 testing. N Engl J Med 2020;383(5):494–6.

21. Hart B, Tu YP, Jennings R, et al. A comparison of health care worker-collected foam and polyester nasal swabs in convalescent COVID-19 patients. PLoS One 2020;15(10):e0241100.

22. Tsang NNY, So HC, Ng KY, et al. Diagnostic performance of different sampling approaches for SARS-CoV-2 RT-PCR testing: a systematic review and meta-analysis. Lancet Infect Dis 2021;21(9):1233–45.

23. LeBlanc JJ, Heinstein C, MacDonald J, et al. A combined oropharyngeal/nares swab is a suitable alternative to nasopharyngeal swabs for the detection of SARS-CoV-2. J Clin Virol 2020;128:104442.

24. Price TK, Bowland BC, Chandrasekaran S, et al. Performance characteristics of severe acute respiratory Syndrome coronavirus 2 RT-PCR tests in a single health system: analysis of >10,000 results from three different Assays. J Mol Diagn 2021;23(2):159–63.

25. Cevik M, Tate M, Lloyd O, et al. SARS-CoV-2, SARS-CoV, and MERS-CoV viral load dynamics, duration of viral shedding, and infectiousness: a systematic review and meta-analysis. Lancet Microbe 2021;2(1):e13–22.

26. Stanoeva KR, van der Eijk AA, Meijer A, et al. Towards a sensitive and accurate interpretation of molecular testing for SARS-CoV-2: a rapid review of 264 studies. Euro Surveill 2021;26(10).

27. Walsh KA, Jordan K, Clyne B, et al. SARS-CoV-2 detection, viral load and infectivity over the course of an infection. J Infect 2020;81(3):357–71.

28. Wolfel R, Corman VM, Guggemos W, et al. Virological assessment of hospitalized patients with COVID-2019. Nature 2020;581(7809):465–9.

29. Zhurakivska K, Troiano G, Pannone G, et al. An Overview of the temporal shedding of SARS-CoV-2 RNA in clinical specimens. Front Public Health 2020;8:487.

30. Zapor M. Persistent detection and infectious potential of SARS-CoV-2 virus in clinical specimens from COVID-19 patients. Viruses 2020;12(12).

31. Wang W, Xu Y, Gao R, et al. Detection of SARS-CoV-2 in different types of clinical specimens. Jama 2020;323(18):1843–4.

32. Huang Y, Chen S, Yang Z, et al. SARS-CoV-2 viral load in clinical samples from Critically ill patients. Am J Respir Crit Care Med 2020;201(11):1435–8.

33. Interim Laboratory CDC. Biosafety guidelines for Handling and processing specimens associated with Coronavirus disease 2019 (COVID-19). 2021. Available at:

https://www.cdc.gov/coronavirus/2019-ncov/lab/lab-biosafety-guidelines.html. Accessed May 2021.

34. Winichakoon P, Chaiwarith R, Liwsrisakun C, et al. Negative nasopharyngeal and oropharyngeal swabs do not Rule out COVID-19. J Clin Microbiol 2020;58(5).

35. Hanson KECA, Arias CA, Hayden MK, et al. Infectious diseases Society of America guidelines on the diagnosis of COVID-19: molecular diagnostic testing. Infectious Diseases Society of America. 2020. *Version 200.* 2020;Available at. https://www.idsociety.org/practice-guideline/covid-19-guideline-diagnostics/. Accessed May 22 2021.

36. Parasa S, Desai M, Thoguluva Chandrasekar V, et al. Prevalence of gastrointestinal symptoms and fecal viral shedding in patients with coronavirus disease 2019: a systematic review and meta-analysis. JAMA Netw Open 2020;3(6): e2011335.

37. Rokkas T. Gastrointestinal involvement in COVID-19: a systematic review and meta-analysis. Ann Gastroenterol 2020;33(4):355–65.

38. van Doorn AS, Meijer B, Frampton CMA, et al. Systematic review with meta-analysis: SARS-CoV-2 stool testing and the potential for faecal-oral transmission. Aliment Pharmacol Ther 2020;52(8):1276–88.

39. National CDC. Wastewater surveillance system (NWSS). 2021. Available at: https://www.cdc.gov/coronavirus/2019-ncov/cases-updates/wastewater-surveillance.html. Accessed May 2021.

40. FDA. Coronavirus Disease 2019 testing Basics. Accessed December 17, 2021. 2021.

41. Fajnzylber J, Regan J, Coxen K, et al. SARS-CoV-2 viral load is associated with increased disease severity and mortality. Nat Commun 2020;11(1):5493.

42. Bakkour S, Saa P, Groves JA, et al. Minipool testing for SARS-CoV-2 RNA in United States blood donors. Transfusion 2021;61(8):2384–91.

43. FDA. Updated Information for Blood Establishments Regarding the COVID-19 Pandemic and Blood Donation. 2021. Available at: https://www.fda.gov/vaccines-blood-biologics/safety-availability-biologics/updated-information-blood-establishments-regarding-covid-19-pandemic-and-blood-donation. Accessed May 23, 2021.

44. Bwire GM, Majigo MV, Njiro BJ, et al. Detection profile of SARS-CoV-2 using RT-PCR in different types of clinical specimens: a systematic review and meta-analysis. J Med Virol 2021;93(2):719–25.

45. Johnson H, Garg M, Shantikumar S, et al. COVID-19 (SARS-CoV-2) in Non-Airborne body fluids: a systematic review & Meta-analysis. Turkish J Urol 2021; 47(2):87–97.

46. Zou X, Chen K, Zou J, et al. Single-cell RNA-seq data analysis on the receptor ACE2 expression reveals the potential risk of different human organs vulnerable to 2019-nCoV infection. Front Med 2020;14(2):185–92.

47. Nasr SH, Kopp JB. COVID-19-Associated collapsing glomerulopathy: an emerging entity. Kidney Int Rep 2020;5(6):759–61.

Strategies for Scaling up SARS-CoV-2 Molecular Testing Capacity

Sanchita Das, MD, Karen M. Frank, MD, PhD*

KEYWORDS

• Automation • Capacity • Molecular testing • Pooling • RT-PCR, SARS-CoV-2

KEY POINTS

• Pooling of specimens successfully expanded SARS-CoV-2 testing capacity during a time of supply shortages.
• Rapid implementation of automation provided additional capacity for testing.
• Sensitivity and specificity were maintained with both pooling and automation.

INTRODUCTION

More than 413 million people have been infected with the severe acute respiratory syndrome coronavirus-2 (SARS-CoV-2) resulting in more than 5.8 million deaths worldwide.[1] Testing for the virus at high volumes has been essential in the battle against the pandemic, yet there continues to be huge variation in the ability of different countries to keep up with their testing needs. The number of tests per confirmed case has varied widely as has the total cumulative cases per country. In March 2020, the United States was averaging 21 tests per confirmed case whereas Taiwan was performing 211 tests per confirmed case. Nearly 1 year later at the beginning of February 2021, the United States was still performing just 12 tests per confirmed case compared with Australia, with 451 tests per confirmed case. Importantly, the overall volume of testing in the United States was quite large, with more than 457 million SARS-CoV-2 tests performed by mid-June 2021.[2] Target populations for testing were highly diverse and included patients being admitted to a hospital or being evaluated in a clinic, asymptomatic individuals at work, or students in educational institutions. In this review, we will address the approaches used to increase the capacity of molecular testing for viral RNA, as this remains an important and challenging problem and the lessons learned in the response to SARS-CoV-2 are applicable to future infectious disease pandemics.

Department of Laboratory Medicine, National Institutes of Health Clinical Center, Bethesda, MD 20892, USA
* Correspondence:
E-mail address: karen.frank@nih.gov

Clin Lab Med 42 (2022) 261–282
https://doi.org/10.1016/j.cll.2022.02.006
0272-2712/22/Published by Elsevier Inc.

Strategies used to scale up testing capacity

The following strategies were used to increase the volume of SARS-CoV-2 testing:

- Pooling
- Diversification of platforms
- Decentralization away from public health laboratories
- Conversion of research laboratories into clinical laboratories
- Maximizing number of samples per plate when supplies were low by adjusting the plate layout
- Production of viral transport media in house
- Use of phosphate-buffered saline instead of viral transport media
- Production of 3D-printed swabs
- Validation of assays with lower number of targets
- Multiplexing and automation
- Applying innovative technologies to COVID-19 diagnostics, such as clustered regularly interspaced short palindromic repeats (CRISPR)-based platforms

We will discuss each of these in turn with a focus on pooling.

POOLING

Pooled testing has been used for many years and is ideally suited for situations in which the prevalence of positive samples for an infectious disease is low enough to result in an overall savings of reagents. Models for optimal pool sizes date back nearly 80 years, and testing of blood donations for HIV and hepatitis are excellent examples of successful pooling strategies.[3] Pooling reduces the expense of testing and conserves scarce reagents, which has been critical during the SARS-CoV-2 pandemic when supplies were limiting the testing capacity in many locations. The advantages of robust pooling can be quite dramatic, reducing the number of tests by 90% in low-risk groups.[4]

The following parameters should be considered when adopting a pooling strategy:

- Pooling method (original specimens vs extracted RNA)
- Pooling algorithm
- Size of pool
- Sensitivity of the pooled test

Pooling Method

Pooling is a testing method that combines specimens from multiple subjects into a pool for a single test. When a pool tests negative, the testing is complete for all individual samples in the pool. If the pool tests positive, further testing is required to identify which specimens led to the pool turning positive. An alternative approach is to perform nucleic acid extraction on all specimens individually and then combine the purified products for amplification and signal detection. Studies evaluating the performance of pooled testing have largely focused on nasopharyngeal or midturbinate specimens, but saliva has also been evaluated and shown to pool successfully.

Several groups have developed modifications to traditional algorithms in their efforts to optimize the efficiency of pooled testing strategies. Volpato and colleagues[5] examined pools of 10 nasopharyngeal swabs and found slightly better sensitivity when pooling specimens before extraction compared with testing pooled RNA after extraction. Sanghani and colleagues[6] proposed using large molecular-weight cutoff centrifugal concentrators to improve sensitivity of pooled samples, but this strategy did not show an increase in sensitivity and the proposed method, which adds a step in the procedure, was not successfully implemented for a laboratory performing high-capacity testing. Conversely, Sawicki and colleagues[7] concentrated pools of 6 or 9 samples using a centrifugal filter before RNA extraction and reported the ability to detect samples with cycle threshold (Ct) values as high as 34.

Another strategy is to pool at the time of collection instead of in the laboratory. A study by Christoff and colleagues reported testing of more than 18,000 individuals by collecting 2 swabs per person, wherein 1 swab was placed in a pooled tube of 16 swabs and the other swab was inserted into a separate tube for individual testing in case the pool turns positive. Although this approach relieves the burden on the laboratory for pooling, it uses twice as many swabs, which were in very short supply at times during the pandemic, and required that tracking of the 16 samples be done by the collection site. The prevalence of SARS-CoV-2 in this study was ~1%, and this group was able to show this approach increased their capacity 4.4-fold, which includes the reflex testing after pool deconvolution.[8] Most studies used pooling of original specimen before extraction and this approach will be discussed further when considering optimal pool size.

Pooling Algorithm

Quite a few publications have described mathematical models for predicting optimal pool size for the SARS-CoV-2 pandemic. One-dimensional pooling, called the Dorfman approach, is the simplest and most commonly used approach. For this strategy, each positive pool must be deconvoluted by retesting each sample included in the pool to identify the infected individuals. In most cases, each pool contains 5 to 10 samples. As an example, Ben-Ami and colleagues[9]. reported a 7.3-fold increase in throughput by pooling groups of 8 specimens to test over 26,000 samples.

Modifications to the Dorfman algorithm include sequential pooling, which is a two-dimensional multistep approach wherein a positive pool is broken into smaller pools for repeat testing. The downside is that each round of testing increases the turnaround time. Another form of two-dimensional pooling is a geometric scheme, also called matrix or tapestry pooling, that offers a theoretic benefit of additional saved time and supplies (**Fig. 1**).[10–12] Matrix pooling uses combinatorial mathematical theory to put each sample in multiple pools, with no 2 samples together in more than 1 pool. This approach permits the identification of the positive samples in the first round, without deconvolution and retesting,[13] but the complexity of this scheme would make manual pooling by a technologist very challenging. Two-dimensional pooling strategies may be feasible with the aid of robotic pipetting instruments, but there are no published reports of successful implementation of this approach to date. Some models have illustrated the advantages of pooling homogeneous groups in a context-sensitive manner, such as staff working in the same office, for maximal efficiency. Although the theoretic benefits are clear, this method would greatly increase the complexity of the preanalytical steps for many laboratory operations and potentially outweigh the benefits in reagent savings.[14] One commentary supported an algorithm of split pooling over the Dorfman algorithm, suggesting that every pool should be tested twice if negative before reporting the negative result; however, this process would lead to unacceptable delays in result reporting. Furthermore, the investigators claim that modern automated laboratory equipment makes it is easy to carry out split pool testing and does not fully capture the complex realities of sample tracking and workflows in the clinical laboratory.[15]

Others have proposed an approach to optimize the testing strategy by considering prevalence and potentially having a different algorithm for a low-risk versus a high-risk

METHOD A - SIMPLE

Round 1: 3 tests of 9 per pool

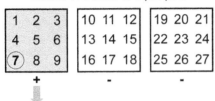

+   -   -

Round 2: 9 tested individually

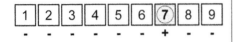

-   -   -   -   -   -   +   -   -

Total tests: **12** for 27 individuals

METHOD B - SEQUENTIAL

Round 1: 3 tests of 9 per pool

+   -   -

Round 2: 3 tests of 3 per pool

| 1 | 2 | 3 | -
| 4 | 5 | 6 | -
| ⑦ | 8 | 9 | +

Round 3: 3 tested individually

| ⑦ | 8 | 9 |
+   -   -

Total tests: **9** for 27 individuals

METHOD C - MATRIX/TAPESTRY

Round 1: 6 tests of 3 per pool
Each sample in >1 pool
Detect positive sample by pattern

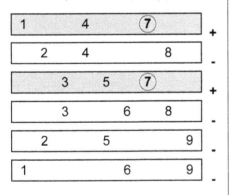

Total tests: **18** for 27 individuals

METHOD D - COMBINATION

Round 1: 3 tests of 9 per pool

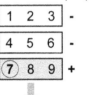

+   -   -

Round 2: 6 tests of 3 per pool (T1-T6)
Each sample in 2 pools
Detect positive sample by pattern

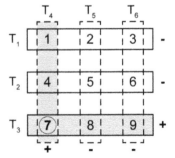

Total tests: **9** for 27 individuals

Fig. 1. Algorithms for pooled testing. The simple method is also called the Dorfman method (A). These show simple examples of only one positive (Sample #7) out of 27 samples tested. Methods C and D, in particular, would be more complex as prevalence increases and pools contain multiple positive samples.

population.[4] However, the rapid changing of procedures on a week-to-week basis must consider the training of technical staff and their ability to adjust to modifications in a procedure without error. Automated programmable pooling on an instrument, when available, would reduce the potential element of human error at that step; however, the challenge of rapidly switching between different preanalytical and postanalytical workflows would remain and likely explains why there are very few examples of rapid shifting of pooling algorithms beyond a simple adjustment of pool size with prevalence. Another proposal has been to group samples for pooling by age, but the advantages were shown to be minuscule relative to the extra burden this approach would place on a laboratory.[16] A table comparing efficiency of the Dorman pooling algorithm versus matrix pooling showed variation with prevalence, with the Dorfman method being favored at a low prevalence and the matrix slightly favored at 10% prevalence.[9] Although modeling remains a very valuable tool for exploring many different pooling strategies, empiric studies that have actually validated and implemented pooling are more valuable than simulations.

Size of Pool

The optimal size of a pool depends on the prevalence of the disease as well as the pooling algorithm. As the number of positive pools increases with rising prevalence, the number of tests performed approaches or exceeds that of standard nonpooling methods, thereby negating the savings that would have been realized through more efficient use of reagents. Thus, although the theoretic benefits of pooling have been demonstrated up to a positivity rate of 30%, at such high levels the pool size would need to be exceedingly small to prevent every pool from testing positive and requiring deconvolution. Pool sizes of 10 are optimal over a broader range of prevalence and most studies recommend pooling only if the prevalence is less than 10%.[17,18] Commonly suggested pool sizes range from 4 to 10, though some studies advocate for 32 to 64 samples per pool (**Table 1**).[7,19–27]

The largest real-world study evaluating the performance of a pooled testing strategy comes from Barak and colleagues, who analyzed 17,945 pools created from 133,816 samples drawn from symptomatic and asymptomatic individuals affiliated with the Hadassah Medical Center in Jerusalem, Israel. The investigators used the Dorfman algorithm with pool sizes of either 5 or 8, depending on the prior week's pool positivity rate. Their use of a dynamic pool size, as well as the nonrandom clustering of positive samples based on the location of testing (nursing homes, colleges, and health care settings), resulted in a 76% reduction in the number of polymerase chain reactions (PCR), which exceeded the predicted performance of their strategy. The investigators note the ability to adjust pool size was facilitated by their use of automated liquid handlers.[28] A study by Petrovan and colleagues[29] reported efficient detection with pools of up to 80 specimens, but the study validated their protocol using only specimens with high viral loads; therefore, conclusions cannot be generalized to settings in which a significant proportion of specimens are expected to have lower viral loads.

Sensitivity of Pooled Testing

A primary concern with combining multiple specimens into a pool is that it will dilute the signal of individual tests, resulting in the missed detection of low viral load specimens. However, nucleic acid amplification tests for viral RNA are highly sensitive, with a limit of detection as low as 5 copies of virus per reaction. This degree of sensitivity is the reason why pooling has been immensely successful for HIV and hepatitis as there is only a minor loss of sensitivity. With SARS-CoV-2, the realization that specimens with low viral loads are often (though not always) associated with a lower transmission

Table 1
Examples of reports of implemented pooled testing of SARS-CoV-2

Type of Pooling	Pool Size	Specimen Type	Assay	Number Tested	Results	Reference
Simple	5, 10, 15, 5 for large volume analysis	NP	Pathofinder Real Accurate Quadruplex Corona-plus PCR Kit	4475 in 895 pools	Ct ↓ by 2.2, Acceptable for Ct 16.7–39.4	Alcoba-Florez et al.[19] 2021
Simple	4	NP MT Nasal	Quest Diagnostics SARS-CoV-2 RNA Qualitative Real-Time RT-PCR	3091	Ct ↓ 1.9/2.38, PPA: 100%	Borillo et al.[20] 2020
Simple	5, 7, 10	NP MT	CDC Assay, Panther Fusion SARS-CoV-2	270, then 7000	Ct ↓ by 2.7–3.6 (10 in pool), 0.2–1.8 (5, 7 in pool), Detected all positives with Ct < 36 for all pool sizes	Das et al.[21] 2020
Simple	6	NP Saliva	Roche Cobas SARS-CoV-2	564	Sensitivity: NP 100%, Saliva 90%; 25% of samples had Ct > 30	McMillen et al.[22] 2021
Simple	5, 10	NP	TaqPath Covid-19 Multiplex Diagnostic Solution	630	Detected Ct 33 consistently for pool of 5, Detected Ct 31 consistently for pool of 10	More et al.[23] 2021
Simple	5, 10	Saliva	Sansure SARS-CoV-2 Nucleic Acid Diagnostic Kit	200	Pools of 5 or 10 acceptable	Pasomsub et al.[24] 2021
Simple	2, 4, 8, 16, 32, 64	Nasal and Throat	AgPath ID One-Step RT-PCR, WHO primer/probe, BioRad CFX96	72	10% False negative rate for pool of 32, Sensitivity for pool of 16: 96%	Yelin et al.[25] 2020

Simple	6, 9	NP, Nasal + OP	Concentrate pool with Amicon Ultra 0.5 mL Ultracell 30K Filter, QIAamp Minicolumn, Z-Path-COVID-19-CE Genesig Real-Time RT-PCR (Primerdesign)	112	Ct decrease 0.5–3, Detected as high as Ct 34	Sawicki et al.[7] 2021
Simple	5, 9	Upper respiratory swab	CDC RT-PCR	20 positives into 60 for pools of 5 and into 39 for pools of 9	For CT ≥ 33, sensitivity 95% for pools of 5% and 87% for pools of 9	Griesemer et al.[36] 2021
Simple	5, 10, 20	Saliva	Luna Universal Probe One-Step RTqPCR, Laboratory Developed primer/probe, Biorad CFX 96 q PCR	23 pools of 5, 23 pools of 10, 31 pools of 20	Sensitivity: 93% for pools of 5%, 89% for pools of 10%, 85% for pools of 20	Watkins et al.[33] 2021
Simple	4, 8	NP	Laboratory-developed assay	320	Sensitivity: 75% for pools of 4, 62.5% for pools of 8	Mahmoud et al.[37] 2021
Simple	5, 8	NP	Laboratory-developed assay QIAsymphony extraction TaqPath Master Mix QuantStudio 5 LiHa Robot	133,816	Adjusted pool size with prevalence of 0.5%–6%. Spared 76% pf reagents	Barak et al.[28] 2021

Abbreviations: positive percent agreement, PPA; nasopharyngeal, NP; mid-turbinate, MT; oropharyngeal, OP; cycle threshold, Ct.

risk paved the way for pooling methods to be accepted by laboratory, hospital, and public health leadership.

Multiple studies have now demonstrated that the slight loss of sensitivity from pooling samplings does not affect the detection of virus from individual samples when they contain RNA levels that correspond to transmissible disease. In most studies this equates to Ct values below 35.[30–32] Importantly, a key decision for an institution is setting the upper bound for Ct value that must be detected in their assay. For example, do specimens with viral loads corresponding to a Ct value of 38 need to be detected, or should only specimens with a Ct value of 34 and lower be considered essential for identification? Ultimately, determining an acceptable loss of sensitivity is a subjective determination of the highest Ct value present in the individuals most likely to spread disease and must be informed by careful epidemiologic studies that are specific to the set of SARS-CoV-2 variants in current circulation.[33]

The key parameter influencing sensitivity is pool size. Wang and colleagues examined a lab-developed test and Panther assays with pools of four reporting a sensitivity of 83%–100% and with pools of eight reporting a sensitivity of 72% to 83%. All false negatives had a Ct value greater than 34.[34] Abdalhamid and colleagues[35] reported that pools of five specimens dropped the highest detectable Ct value of an individual specimen by 0 to 5 cycles although it also reduced the number of tests performed by 69%. Griesemer and colleagues[36] showed pooling of five specimens detected 95% of individual positive samples, but pools of nine detected only 87%. This group focused on identifying samples with Ct values of 33 to 36. Watkins and colleagues[33] reported a sensitivities of 93%, 89%, and 85% for saliva pool sizes of 5, 10, and 20, respectively. A study by Mahmoud and colleagues[37] reported high false negative rates with pools of 4 and 8, but this result was not typical, as the investigators noted difficulty identifying positive samples with a Ct value > 30 whereas many other studies show good sensitivity detecting samples with Ct values as high as 34.

Regulation

From the beginning of the pandemic, the United States Food and Drug Administration (FDA) regulated testing for SARS-CoV-2 for both commercial and laboratory-developed tests because of the potential public health consequences of poor-quality tests used on a massive scale. Early FDA guidance limited pool size to 4 to 8 specimens, even though models suggested that larger pool sizes when deployed in low-prevalence settings would remain effective.[38,39] The recommendations have been since relaxed, but the validation studies require extensive documentation on expected changes in sensitivity, handling of PCR inhibitors, and deconvolution methods.

Preanalytical/Postanalytical Considerations

When properly calibrated to prevalence, pooled testing strategies result in significant savings. However, this comes at the cost of increased preanalytical and postanalytical complexity. Specimen handling becomes more challenging as the pools must be made by an instrument or a technologist. Uncapping and recapping tubes can become a limiting factor for some automated workflows. Furthermore, the larger the pool size, the higher the risk of a specimen mix-up at the time of deconvolution.

A limitation of pooling is that it removes the ability to assess for individual sampling adequacy through a positive internal control, such as the human RNAse P gene. However, our experience has been that the rate of inadequate samples was extremely low for nasopharyngeal, midturbinate, and saliva collections; therefore, this is not likely to be a major drawback. It should be noted that pooling does not reduce the workload for reporting and billing and instead has increased the work for the information technology staff who must create new data management algorithms for result reporting.[40]

Summary of Pooling

Many laboratories have successfully implemented robust pooling algorithms to efficiently scale up SARS-CoV-2 molecular testing. Lessons learned from the current pandemic will serve to inform laboratories that may need rapid scale-up of testing in the future.

NEED FOR SCALE-UP OF MOLECULAR ASSAYS FOR SARS-CoV-2

Highly sensitive reverse transcriptase-PCR (RT-PCR) testing and contact tracing has been the cornerstone of containment strategies during the pandemic but is predicated on the ability to return accurate results as fast as possible. Mathematical modeling showed that testing delays of more than 3 days significantly reduces the prevention of transmission by contact tracing.[41] Recognizing the need for expanded capacity of rapid testing, initiatives such as the NIH RADx were developed early in the pandemic to speed development of new tests.[42] These and other studies recognized several challenges that would need to be overcome before large scale testing could be instituted.

Challenges to implementation of RT-PCR–based large-scale testing include the availability of high-throughput assays and platforms, adequate access to sufficient reagents, laboratory infrastructure, and the ability for laboratories to develop and validate new assays, the availability of trained personnel and the costs of implementing high capacity population-based testing strategies.[43–45] We consider several strategies to overcome these challenges in the following sections.

STRATEGIES TO CONSIDER FOR LARGE-SCALE TESTING FOR SARS-CoV-2
Increase in Testing Capacity by Modification of Traditional Laboratory-Developed Tests

One of the simplest means of increasing testing capacity is to increase the use of automated RNA extraction methods. Indeed, global shortages and bottlenecks in production of extraction reagents prompted an assortment of studies that investigated alternate extraction procedures or direct PCR amplification on specimens.[20,46] Several studies have evaluated the use of liquid handling robots, describing methods to increase efficiency while reducing dependency on commercial kits. Lazaro-Perona and colleagues evaluated an in-house developed liquid handling system (OT-2) and compared its performance with that of the MagMAX (ThermoFisher Scientific) commercial kit-based extraction platform. The Ct values for the *orf1ab* and S gene targets from clinical specimens were comparable between the 2 methods. The robot required intensive programming that was shared on an open access repository.[47] Borillo and colleagues evaluated a Tecan Evo 150 automated liquid handler (Tecan Group Limited, Männedorf, Switzerland) using the PHASIFY viral RNA extraction kit (PHASE Scientific International Ltd., Hong Kong). This method was found to be superior to extraction using the NucliSENS easyMAG (bioMérieux, Marcy-l'Étoile, France), especially for saliva specimens.[20]

Another simple and effective method to scale up testing would be to remove the extraction procedure altogether by performing RT-PCR directly on the specimen or on minimally processed specimens. Although this strategy does not actually automate the procedure or increase throughput, it does reduce hands-on labor and time while bypassing the reagent supply chain shortages. The key objectives of an extraction procedure, inactivation of virus and release of RNA, can be achieved by a simple heat inactivation step in the presence of proteinase K as shown by Vogels and colleagues[48] in their SalivaDirect method. Their nucleic acid extraction-free method was successful in detecting SARS-CoV-2 RNA using a dualplex RT-PCR assay with 6 to 12 RNA copies/μL using reagents from multiple vendors. Additional advantages of SalivaDirect were the low supply cost and the stability of the specimen for up to 7 days without compromise in sensitivity. Claas and colleagues[49] evaluated the combination of an automated liquid handling robot, the Tecan Fluent 480 (Tecan Switzerland), with a simplified commercial liquid sample preparation for direct RT-PCR and showed acceptable sensitivity and specificity in SARS-CoV-2 samples with Ct values of less than 33. Use of detergents and guanidinium isothiocyanate with chloroform for direct sample preparation showed variable sensitivity. Of note, some of these studies demonstrated a loss of sensitivity when detergents or other extraction reagents or heat inactivation methods were used in direct sample preparation in RT-PCR.[50–52] Caution and proper biosafety precautions should also be used when using these non-extraction sample preparations to determine the level of viral inactivation.[49,53]

Combining methods to reduce extraction steps and multiplexing several probes in a single reaction is also an effective way of increasing capacity. An additional advantage of multiplexed assays is panel testing that includes other respiratory viral targets. This would significantly increase testing efficiency during the respiratory viral season when influenza or respiratory syncytial virus may be circulating and patients may have similar symptoms early in the disease. Several laboratories validated a multiplexed version of the available SARS-CoV-2 assays before implementation of the assay in clinical care during the initial phases of the pandemic to reduce consumption of resources.[54,55] A newer version of the CDC SARS-CoV-2 assay that received FDA authorization for emergency use in January 2021 is a multiplexed assay for detection of influenza A and B along with SARS-CoV-2 across a broad range of instruments that permit high-throughput extraction. Shortly thereafter, multiplexed commercial assays for respiratory pathogens such as the BioFire Respiratory 2.1 Panel and Xpert Xpress CoV-2/Flu/RSV (Cepheid, Sunnyvale, CA) received FDA authorization and provide rapid actionable results during respiratory season.

Increase in Testing Capacity Using Automated Platforms

As the capacity required to meet demand increased to millions of tests per day, it became clear that the need for reagents and labor would far exceeded the available global supply chain. Automated platforms are capable of significantly increasing throughput while reducing human error and achieving high diagnostic precision. Such platforms have been meaningful during past outbreaks such as Ebola, Zika, and HIV.[42] From these past experiences, we have learned that an ideal diagnostic platform is low complexity, high throughput, random access, able to detect multiple targets in a single run, have limited need for human labor, and occupy a small floor area. There are several FDA-approved high-throughput automated platforms that offer large-scale testing for SARS-CoV-2[56], however, one that satisfies all of the above conditions, while also being affordable and devoid of supply chain issues, does not exist. Most of the existing platforms combine nucleic acid extraction, amplification, detection, analysis, and reporting of results, thus increasing throughput, accuracy, and precision while reducing sources of human error at both analytical and postanalytical steps. The performance characteristics are comparable as shown in recent studies (**Table 2**), but there are differences in the functionality of these platforms, including throughput per 8-h work shift, technician hands-on time, and random-access capability. Many clinical laboratories use multiple platforms simultaneously to efficiently

Table 2

Example of investigations of clinical performance of fully automated platforms for the detection of SARS-CoV-2

Platform(s) Evaluated	Study Design	Type and Number of Specimens	Comparator Method	Results of Study	Reference
Hologic Panther Fusion SARS-CoV-2 Assay (Fusion) Hologic Aptima SARS-CoV-2 Assay (Aptima) BioFire Defense COVID-19 test (Biofire)	Retrospective and prospective	Nasopharyngeal swab (n = 150)	Consensus results from 3 platforms	94.7%–98.7% PPA, 100% NPA	Smith et al.[83] 2020
Hologic Panther Fusion SARS-CoV-2 Assay (Fusion) Simplexa COVID-19 Direct (Diasorin) assay GenMark ePlex SARS-CoV-2 (GenMark) assay	Retrospective and prospective	Nasopharyngeal swab (n = 104)	CDC SARS-CoV-2 assay	96%–100% PPA and NPA	Zhen et al.[84] 2020
Hologic Panther Fusion SARS-CoV-2 assay (Fusion) cobas SARS-CoV-2 RT-PCR using cobas 6800 system	Retrospective and prospective	Nasopharyngeal swab (n = 389)	Comparison of 2 platforms and Xpert Xpress SARS-CoV-2 RT-PCR for discrepancy analysis	96.4% agreement in performance	Craney et al.[85] 2020
RealTime SARS-CoV-2 assay using m2000 system (Abbott)	Validation and verification	Nasal and nasopharyngeal swab (n = 30)	Comparison to CDC SARS-CoV-2 assay	Sensitivity 93% Specificity 100%	Degli-Angeli et al.[86] 2020
RealTime SARS-CoV-2 assay using Alinity m system (Abbott) cobas SARS-CoV-2 RT-PCR using cobas 6800 system (Roche)	Prospective	Nasopharyngeal swab (n = 2129)	Clinical evaluation of performance	100% PPA,96.8% NPA	Kogoj et al.[87] 2021

(continued on next page)

Table 2
(continued)

Platform(s) Evaluated	Study Design	Type and Number of Specimens	Comparator Method	Results of Study	Reference
NeuMoDx 96 Molecular System (Ann Arbor, MI)	Retrospective (stored for < 5 d)	Nasopharyngeal swab (n = 159)	Comparison of NeuMoDx to Diasorin Simplexa SARS-CoV-2 direct assay and CDC SARS-CoV-2 assay	100% PPA and NPA	Lima et al.[88] 2020
NeuMoDx 96 Molecular System (Ann Arbor, MI)	Multicenter comparison, retrospective	Nasopharyngeal swab (n = 212)	New York SARS-CoV-2 Real-time Reverse Transcriptase (RT)-PCR Diagnostic Panel and RealStar® SARS-CoV-2 RT-PCR Kit 1.0 (Altona Diagnostics, Hamburg, Germany)	99% PPA, 91.5% NPA	Mostafa et al.[89] 2020

Abbreviations: NPA, negative percent agreement; PPA, positive percent agreement.

increase testing capacity while maintaining flexibility to satisfy a wide range of clinical needs. **Table 3** summarizes the factors that may be considered by the laboratory before implementing these expensive platforms.

Alternative Technologies for Diagnosis

Diversification of technologies can also aid in the scale up of testing, especially given the concerns with reagent availability and supply chain issues. Several new technologies have been developed during the pandemic that can be implemented in large-scale testing.

CRISPR and associated Cas protein-based diagnostics are powerful methods for nucleic acid detection using cleavage activity. These are typically used in conjunction with reverse transcription loop-mediated isothermal amplification (RT-LAMP) and other isothermal methods. The assays SHERLOCK AND DETECTR have been

Table 3
Factors to consider before acquisition of automated platforms for high-throughput assays during a time of crisis

Goal	Key Parameters to be Assessed	Other Factors
Is this the right assay for this disease?	• Clinical condition being tested • Specimen types or matrix that will be tested • Instrument turnaround time	Clinical and analytical performance characteristics of assay: • Sensitivity • Specificity • Lower limit of detection • Positive and negative predictive values
Is this the appropriate instrument for this test?	• Throughput of instrument (number of tests per 8-h shift) • Hands-on time required before specimen is loaded on the instrument • Availability of reagents, compatibility with commercial reagents	• Batch tested vs random access • Available staffing • Backup plans to mitigate risks for reagent or supply shortages
Is this the appropriate instrument for my laboratory?	• Cost of the instrument and cost per assay • Price of maintenance and repairs • Compatibility with existing testing protocols used in the laboratory • Adaptability to future tests that may be introduced to the laboratory • Instrument footprint	• 5-y return on investment • Service contract costs • Downtime associated with maintenance • Capability to transition laboratory-developed assays to the automated platform • Assessment of assays that are in development for this instrument and whether they fit in with the future plan of the laboratory • Available laboratory space • Need for current or future construction

validated on clinical specimens and are based on cleavage of reporter RNA molecules by the Cas12/13 enzymes.[57] They are available in lateral flow and fluorescence-based readouts and have also been adapted for direct testing of specimens. Further modification of the RNA extraction step by using magnetic beads in conjunction with CRISPR-based assay has been used to expedite detection of SARS-CoV-2 RNA in a "one-pot" test.[58–60] A platform for rapidly scalable diagnostic testing with multiplexing capability has been described by Ackerman and colleagues[61] in the CARMEN-Cas13 assay design. This immensely scalable platform is based on the CRISPR-Cas13 detection system and applied in a combinatorial plate-based format to increase throughput and multiplexing capability.

Nanotechnology is another option that could reduce reagent cost. Use of magnetic nanoparticles for RNA extraction can significantly scale up diagnostic testing and has been advocated for areas with limited resources.[62] The small size and photostability of quantum dots and gold nanoparticles have been used in a colorimetric assay to detect SARS-CoV-2 nucleocapsid gene RNA. Another example is a clinical diagnostic biosensor molecule using gold nanoislands, which can precisely detect selected SARS-CoV-2 sequences in a multigene mixture with low false positive rates.[63,64] Finally, biosensors using graphene–gold nanoparticle platforms can generate an electric readout that was found to be highly sensitive and accurate with rapid turn-around time.[65]

Isothermal amplification techniques such as RT-LAMP have been investigated to ramp up testing as they do not require thermal amplification and therefore the need to transport specimens to a centralized laboratory. They are also amenable to testing crude samples as they are agnostic to PCR inhibitors. Use of multiple primers increases the versatility of these assays in multiplexed reactions. The major disadvantage of the isothermal techniques is the lower sensitivity and specificity when compared with RT-PCR and the requirement for significant optimization for performance comparable to conventional RT-PCR. Several iterations of these assays have been developed in the form of lateral flow or biosensor-based platforms for use in large scale testing at entry points, after addressing the performance characteristics.[66–68]

Although systems like CARMEN have the theoretic potential to perform thousands of assays during a single 8-h shift, most clinical laboratories have been performing the bulk of their testing on commercial automated platforms that use modifications of conventional RT-PCR assays. The newer techniques remain in the research realm because of several challenges and bottlenecks associated with deploying a new assay into a clinical laboratory in the middle of a public health crisis. These include but are not limited to regulatory compliance, complexity of the assays, and adaptability to the CLIA-certified laboratory. Finally, the biggest bottleneck is finding commercial partners such that the reagent and consumable supply chain can be maintained as long as enhanced testing capacity is required.

Next-Generation Sequencing Large-Scale Surveillance of SARS-CoV-2

The need to understand the route of transmission, phylogeny, and molecular evolution of the virus was appreciated early in the pandemic. The emergence of more transmissible variants of SARS-CoV-2 or those that evade immunity induced by vaccines have prompted the development of novel therapeutics. The changing landscape of viral variants underscore the need to monitor their evolution in real-time.[69] Global surveillance efforts (such as COGUK)[70] and sharing of genome sequences in publicly available databases (GISAID)[71] has made an immense impact in efforts to understand the evolution and spread of the viral mutants as well as in studying the immune response to vaccines.[72] Several commercial assays based on NGS have been adapted to high-throughput formats. These platforms can provide comprehensive information about viral genomes for thousands of individuals in a single run.[73,74] Another important role played by NGS is the monitoring and surveillance of environmental samples, such as wastewater for SARS-CoV-2.[75] Levels of viral RNA in these samples have been shown to increase and decrease ahead of case counts making their monitoring useful for early warning systems, including for the detection of variants of concern.[76] Rapid, multiplexed RT-PCR based assays that detect mutations defining variants of concern have been described for both surveillance and screening.[77–79]

LIMITATIONS OF MOLECULAR ASSAYS AND FUTURE STRATEGIES FOR LARGE-SCALE TESTING

As newer technologies and innovative platforms are introduced to laboratories world-wide, strategies must be developed to expeditiously remove the bottlenecks of

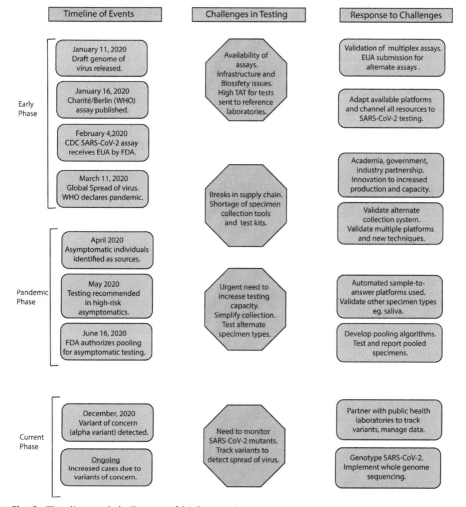

Fig. 2. Timeline and challenges of high-capacity testing. TAT, Turnaround time.

standardization and validation globally. Maintenance of quality control of reagents will be important in deployment of assays. Industry partnership and collaboration with local regulatory authorities will need to be planned.[80] Most importantly, continuous maintenance of the global supply chain is needed to sustain testing capacity.

Another important limitation is that the performance of RT-PCR and other molecular assays have been variable based on the specimen source. Early in the pandemic, lower respiratory swab specimens were reported to be more sensitive in detecting low viral copy numbers than upper respiratory tract specimens.[35] Alternate specimen types such as saliva and oropharyngeal swabs were extremely useful in diagnostic and surveillance testing whereas stool, urine, and blood were not deemed to have sufficient sensitivity to be of use. This variation of detectable RNA quantity in specimen sources will continue to affect the sensitivity and specificity of assays that are being developed. Carefully done studies comparing test performance by body site of collection using standardized gold standards are essential for informing testing algorithms and will become increasingly important if a virus evolves to have new tissue tropism. In addition, RT-PCR assays do not provide essential information regarding viability of the virus.

As with many molecular assays for RNA viruses, continuous monitoring of the performance of primers and probes is required as mutations accrue because of the natural evolution of the virus in response to immune selective pressures and other forces. Significant mutations in the primer/probe binding sites can alter the performance of an assay, thus affecting diagnosis and control efforts. FDA monitors SARS-CoV-2 mutations for possible impact on assay performance,[81] but clinical laboratories are often the first place that changes in analytical performance are noted because of their close involvement with clinicians treating patients with COVID-19. The need to scale up genomic surveillance to detect viral mutants will continue to remain a challenge in the near future.[82] A summary of the challenges of high-capacity testing is shown in **Fig. 2**.

SUMMARY

Clinical laboratories have stepped up to the unprecedented challenges brought on by the COVID-19 pandemic. Although sufficient testing was not available during the initial weeks of the pandemic, multiple strategies were successfully used to address the challenge of extremely high-capacity testing with reliable results. Although many approaches to pooling were proposed, the simple Dorfman algorithm of combining 4 to 10 original specimens before extraction is the most frequently used. Traditional RT-PCR platforms evolved from low-throughput laboratory developed assays to emergency-use authorized commercial assays on high-throughput platforms. However, the diversification of platforms only partially alleviated the supply shortages that persisted for many months. These challenges spurred the development of many innovative technologies such as highly multiplexed CRISPR-based assays although these remain largely in the research and public health realm. As the virus continually evolves, clinical laboratories must remain vigilant and work closely with state and federal public health agencies to ensure the fidelity of their large-scale testing algorithms and platforms remains intact.

CLINICS CARE POINTS

- Multiple strategies for pooling of different types specimens provided sensitive and specific SARS-CoV-2 testing.

- Automated liquid handling, alternative extraction procedures, multiplexing, and rapid commercialization of new testing platforms added to overall testing capacity.
- Innovation of molecular methods, such as CRISPR-based assays, diversified options for testing and also increased overall testing capacity.

DISCLOSURE

The authors have nothing to disclose.

ACKNOWLEDGMENTS

We thank Erica Frank for assistance with the development of **Fig. 1**. This work was supported by the Intramural Research Programs of the National Institutes of Health Clinical Center. This review presents the views of the authors and does not necessarily represent the official positions of the National Institutes of Health or the Department of Health and Human Services.

REFERENCES

1. Dong E, Du H, Gardner L. An interactive web-based dashboard to track COVID-19 in real time. Lancet Infect Dis 2020;20(5):533–4.
2. Rosner M, Ritchie H, Ortiz-Ospina E, et al. Coronavirus pandemic (COVID-19). Available at: https://ourworldindata.org/coronavirus. accessed 06/19/2021.
3. Dorfman R. The detection of defective members of large populations. Ann Math Stat 1943;14:436–40.
4. Bish DR, Bish EK, El-Hajj H, et al. A robust pooled testing approach to expand COVID-19 screening capacity. PLoS One 2021;16(2):e0246285.
5. Volpato F, Lima-Morales D, Wink PL, et al. Pooling of samples to optimize SARS-CoV-2 diagnosis by RT-qPCR: comparative analysis of two protocols. Eur J Clin Microbiol Infect Dis 2021;40(4):889–92.
6. Sanghani HR, Nawrot DA, Marmolejo-Cossio F, et al. Concentrating Pooled COVID-19 patient lysates to improve reverse transcription quantitative PCR sensitivity and efficiency. Clin Chem 2021;67(5):797–8.
7. Sawicki R, Korona-Glowniak I, Boguszewska A, et al. Sample pooling as a strategy for community monitoring for SARS-CoV-2. Sci Rep 2021;11(1):3122.
8. Christoff AP, Cruz GNF, Sereia AFR, et al. Swab pooling: a new method for large-scale RT-qPCR screening of SARS-CoV-2 avoiding sample dilution. PLoS One 2021;16(2):e0246544.
9. Ben-Ami R, Klochendler A, Seidel M, et al. Large-scale implementation of pooled RNA extraction and RT-PCR for SARS-CoV-2 detection. Clin Microbiol Infect 2020; 26(9):1248–53.
10. Lagopati N, Tsioli P, Mourkioti I, et al. Sample pooling strategies for SARS-CoV-2 detection. J Virol Methods 2021;289:114044.
11. Millioni R, Mortarino C. Test groups, not individuals: a review of the pooling approaches for SARS-CoV-2 diagnosis. Diagnostics (Basel) 2021;11(1):68.
12. Mallapaty S. The mathematical strategy that could transform coronavirus testing. Nature 2020;583(7817):504–5.
13. Gopalkrishnan M, Krishna S. Pooling samples to increase SARS-CoV-2 Testing. J Indian Inst Sci 2020;100(4):787–92.
14. Deckert A, Barnighausen T, Kyei NN. Simulation of pooled-sample analysis strategies for COVID-19 mass testing. Bull World Health Organ 2020;98(9):590–8.

15. Litvak E, Dentzer S, Pagano M. The right kind of pooled testing for the novel coronavirus: first, do no harm. Am J Public Health 2020;110(12):1772–3.

16. Fernandez-Salinas J, Aragon-Caqueo D, Valdes G, et al. Modelling pool testing for SARS-CoV-2: addressing heterogeneity in populations. Epidemiol Infect 2020;149:e9.

17. Ben-Amotz D. Optimally pooled viral testing. Epidemics 2020;33:100413.

18. Hanel R, Thurner S. Boosting test efficiency by pooled testing for SARS-CoV-2—Formula for optimal pool size. PLoS One 2020;15(11):e0240652.

19. Alcoba-Florez J, Gil-Campesino H, Garcia-Martinez de Artola D, et al. Increasing SARS-CoV-2 RT-qPCR testing capacity by sample pooling. Int J Infect Dis 2021; 103:19–22.

20. Borillo GA, Kagan RM, Baumann RE, et al. Pooling of upper respiratory specimens using a SARS-CoV-2 real-time RT-PCR assay authorized for emergency use in low-prevalence populations for high-throughput testing. Open Forum Infect Dis 2020;7(11):ofaa466.

21. Das S, Lau AF, Youn JH, et al. Pooled testing for surveillance of SARS-CoV-2 in asymptomatic individuals. J Clin Virol 2020;132:104619.

22. McMillen T, Jani K, Babady NE. Evaluation of sample pooling for SARS-CoV-2 RNA detection in nasopharyngeal swabs and saliva on the Roche Cobas 6800. J Clin Virol 2021;138:104790.

23. More S, Narayanan S, Patil G, et al. Pooling of nasopharyngeal swab samples to overcome a global shortage of real-time reverse transcription-PCR COVID-19 test kits. J Clin Microbiol 2021;59(4):e01295-20.

24. Pasomsub E, Watcharananan SP, Watthanachockchai T, et al. Saliva sample pooling for the detection of SARS-CoV-2. J Med Virol 2021;93(3):1506–11.

25. Yelin I, Aharony N, Tamar ES, et al. Evaluation of COVID-19 RT-qPCR test in multi sample pools. Clin Infect Dis 2020;71(16):2073–8.

26. Pikovski A, Bentele K. Pooling of coronavirus tests under unknown prevalence. Epidemiol Infect 2020;148:e183.

27. Deka S, Kalita D. Effectiveness of sample pooling strategies for SARS-CoV-2 mass screening by RT-PCR: a scoping review. J Lab Physicians 2020;12(3): 212–8.

28. Barak N, Ben-Ami R, Sido T, et al. Lessons from applied large-scale pooling of 133,816 SARS-CoV-2 RT-PCR tests. Sci Transl Med 2021;13(589):eabf2823.

29. Petrovan V, Vrajmasu V, Bucur AC, et al. Evaluation of commercial qPCR Kits for detection of SARS-CoV-2 in pooled samples. Diagnostics (Basel) 2020;10(7):472.

30. Huang CG, Lee KM, Hsiao MJ, et al. Culture-based virus isolation to evaluate potential infectivity of clinical specimens tested for COVID-19. J Clin Microbiol 2020; 58(8):e01068-20.

31. La Scola B, Le Bideau M, Andreani J, et al. Viral RNA load as determined by cell culture as a management tool for discharge of SARS-CoV-2 patients from infectious disease wards. Eur J Clin Microbiol Infect Dis 2020;39(6):1059–61.

32. Singanayagam A, Patel M, Charlett A, et al. Duration of infectiousness and correlation with RT-PCR cycle threshold values in cases of COVID-19, England, January to May 2020. Euro Surveill 2020;25(32):2001483.

33. Watkins AE, Fenichel EP, Weinberger DM, et al. Increased SARS-CoV-2 testing capacity with pooled saliva samples. Emerg Infect Dis 2021;27(4):1184–7.

34. Wang H, Hogan CA, Miller JA, et al. Performance of nucleic acid amplification tests for detection of severe acute respiratory syndrome Coronavirus 2 in prospectively pooled specimens. Emerg Infect Dis 2021;27(1):92–103.

35. Abdalhamid B, Bilder CR, McCutchen EL, et al. Assessment of specimen pooling to conserve SARS CoV-2 testing resources. Am J Clin Pathol 2020;153(6):715–8.
36. Griesemer SB, Van Slyke G, St George K. Assessment of sample pooling for clinical SARS-CoV-2 Testing. J Clin Microbiol 2021;59(4).
37. Mahmoud SA, Ibrahim E, Thakre B, et al. Evaluation of pooling of samples for testing SARS-CoV- 2 for mass screening of COVID-19. BMC Infect Dis 2021; 21(1):360.
38. Pilcher CD. A data-driven rationale for high-throughput SARS-CoV-2 mass screening programs. JAMA Netw Open 2020;3(12):e2031577.
39. US Food & Drug Administration. Coronavirus (COVID-19) update: FDA issues first emergency authorization for sample pooling in diagnostic testing. 2020. Available at: https://www.fda.gov/news-events/press-announcements/coronavirus-covid-19-update-fda-issues-first-emergency-authorization-sample-pooling-diagnostic. accessed 6/16/21.
40. McKeeby JW, Siwy CM, Revoir J, et al. Unveiling the silent threat among us: leveraging health information technology in the search for asymptomatic COVID 19 healthcare workers. J Am Med Inform Assoc 2021;28(2):377–83.
41. Kretzschmar ME, Rozhnova G, Bootsma MCJ, et al. Impact of delays on effectiveness of contact tracing strategies for COVID-19: a modelling study. Lancet Public Health 2020;5(8):e452–9.
42. Tromberg BJ, Schwetz TA, Perez-Stable EJ, et al. Rapid scaling up of Covid-19 diagnostic testing in the United States - the NIH RADx initiative. N Engl J Med 2020;383(11):1071–7.
43. Giri B, Pandey S, Shrestha R, et al. Review of analytical performance of COVID-19 detection methods. Anal Bioanal Chem 2021;413(1):35–48.
44. Mercer TR, Salit M. Testing at scale during the COVID-19 pandemic. Nat Rev Genet 2021;22(7):415–26.
45. Weissleder R, Lee H, Ko J, et al. COVID-19 diagnostics in context. Sci Transl Med 2020;12(546):eabc1931.
46. Fomsgaard AS, Rosenstierne MW. An alternative workflow for molecular detection of SARS-CoV-2 - escape from the NA extraction kit-shortage, Copenhagen, Denmark, March 2020. Euro Surveill 2020;25(14):2000398.
47. Lazaro-Perona F, Rodriguez-Antolin C, Alguacil-Guillen M, et al, Group, S. A.-C.-W. Evaluation of two automated low-cost RNA extraction protocols for SARS-CoV-2 detection. PLoS One 2021;16(2):e0246302.
48. Vogels CBF, Watkins AE, Harden CA, et al. SalivaDirect: a simplified and flexible platform to enhance SARS-CoV-2 testing capacity. Med (N Y) 2021;2(3): 263–280 e6.
49. Claas ECJ, Smit PW, van Bussel M, et al. A two minute liquid based sample preparation for rapid SARS-CoV2 real-time PCR screening: a multicentre evaluation. J Clin Virol 2021;135:104720.
50. Fassy J, Lacoux C, Leroy S, et al. Versatile and flexible microfluidic qPCR test for high-throughput SARS-CoV-2 and cellular response detection in nasopharyngeal swab samples. PLoS One 2021;16(4):e0243333.
51. Kalnina L, Mateu-Regue A, Oerum S, et al. A simple, safe and sensitive method for SARS-CoV-2 inactivation and RNA extraction for RT-qPCR. APMIS 2021; 129(7):393–400.
52. Maricic T, Nickel O, Aximu-Petri A, et al. A direct RT-qPCR approach to test large numbers of individuals for SARS-CoV-2. PLoS One 2020;15(12):e0244824.
53. Fukumoto T, Iwasaki S, Fujisawa S, et al. Efficacy of a novel SARS-CoV-2 detection kit without RNA extraction and purification. Int J Infect Dis 2020;98:16–7.

54. Park M, Won J, Choi BY, et al. Optimization of primer sets and detection protocols for SARS-CoV-2 of coronavirus disease 2019 (COVID-19) using PCR and real-time PCR. Exp Mol Med 2020;52(6):963–77.

55. Perchetti GA, Nalla AK, Huang ML, et al. Multiplexing primer/probe sets for detection of SARS-CoV-2 by qRT-PCR. J Clin Virol 2020;129:104499.

56. Chen C, Gao G, Xu Y, et al. SARS-CoV-2-positive sputum and feces after conversion of pharyngeal samples in patients with COVID-19. Ann Intern Med 2020; 172(12):832–4.

57. Kevadiya BD, Machhi J, Herskovitz J, et al. Diagnostics for SARS-CoV-2 infections. Nat Mater 2021;20(5):593–605.

58. Broughton JP, Deng X, Yu G, et al. CRISPR-Cas12-based detection of SARS-CoV-2. Nat Biotechnol 2020;38(7):870–4.

59. Joung J, Ladha A, Saito M, et al. Detection of SARS-CoV-2 with SHERLOCK one-pot testing. N Engl J Med 2020;383(15):1492–4.

60. Patchsung M, Jantarug K, Pattama A, et al. Clinical validation of a Cas13-based assay for the detection of SARS-CoV-2 RNA. Nat Biomed Eng 2020;4(12):1140–9.

61. Ackerman CM, Myhrvold C, Thakku SG, et al. Massively multiplexed nucleic acid detection with Cas13. Nature 2020;582(7811):277–82.

62. Chacon-Torres JC, Reinoso C, Navas-Leon DG, et al. Optimized and scalable synthesis of magnetic nanoparticles for RNA extraction in response to developing countries' needs in the detection and control of SARS-CoV-2. Sci Rep 2020;10(1): 19004.

63. Moitra P, Alafeef M, Dighe K, et al. Selective naked-eye detection of SARS-CoV-2 mediated by N gene targeted antisense oligonucleotide capped plasmonic nanoparticles. ACS Nano 2020;14(6):7617–27.

64. Qiu G, Gai Z, Tao Y, et al. Dual-functional plasmonic photothermal biosensors for highly accurate severe acute respiratory syndrome coronavirus 2 detection. ACS Nano 2020;14(5):5268–77.

65. Alafeef M, Dighe K, Moitra P, et al. Rapid, ultrasensitive, and quantitative detection of SARS-CoV-2 using antisense oligonucleotides directed electrochemical biosensor chip. ACS Nano 2020;14:17028–45.

66. Augustine R, Hasan A, Das S, et al. Loop-mediated isothermal amplification (LAMP): a rapid, sensitive, specific, and cost-effective point-of-care test for coronaviruses in the context of COVID-19 pandemic. Biology (Basel) 2020;9(8):182.

67. Ganguli A, Mostafa A, Berger J, et al. Reverse transcription loop-mediated isothermal amplification assay for ultrasensitive detection of SARS-CoV-2 in Saliva and viral transport medium clinical samples. Anal Chem 2021;93(22): 7797–807.

68. Zhu X, Wang X, Han L, et al. Multiplex reverse transcription loop-mediated isothermal amplification combined with nanoparticle-based lateral flow biosensor for the diagnosis of COVID-19. Biosens Bioelectron 2020;166:112437.

69. Meredith LW, Hamilton WL, Warne B, et al. Rapid implementation of SARS-CoV-2 sequencing to investigate cases of health-care associated COVID-19: a prospective genomic surveillance study. Lancet Infect Dis 2020;20(11):1263–71.

70. consortiumcontact@cogconsortium.uk C-GU. An integrated national scale SARS-CoV-2 genomic surveillance network. Lancet Microbe 2020;1(3):e99–100.

71. Elbe S, Buckland-Merrett G. Data, disease and diplomacy: GISAID's innovative contribution to global health. Glob Chall 2017;1(1):33–46.

72. Harvey WT, Carabelli AM, Jackson B, et al. SARS-CoV-2 variants, spike mutations and immune escape. Nat Rev Microbiol 2021;19(7):409–24.

73. Aynaud MM, Hernandez JJ, Barutcu S, et al. A multiplexed, next generation sequencing platform for high-throughput detection of SARS-CoV-2. Nat Commun 2021;12(1):1405.
74. Li T, Chung HK, Pireku PK, et al. Rapid high-throughput whole-genome sequencing of SARS-CoV-2 by using one-step reverse transcription-PCR amplification with an integrated microfluidic system and next-generation sequencing. J Clin Microbiol 2021;59(5):e02784-20.
75. Daughton CG. Wastewater surveillance for population-wide Covid-19: the present and future. Sci Total Environ 2020;736:139631.
76. Kirby AE, Welsh RM, Marsh ZA, Yu AT, Vugia DJ, Boehm AB, Wolfe MK, White BJ, Matzinger SR, Wheeler A, Bankers L, Andresen K, Salatas C, New York City Department of Environmental Protection, Gregory DA, Johnson MC, Trujillo M, Kannoly S, Smyth DS, Dennehy JJ, Sapoval N, Ensor K, Treangen T, Stadler LB, Hopkins L. Notes from the field: early evidence of the SARS-CoV-2 B.1.1.529 (omicron) variant in community wastewater - United States, november-december 2021. MMWR Morb Mortal Wkly Rep 2022;71(3):103–5.
77. Borsova K, Paul ED, Kovacova V, et al. Surveillance of SARS-CoV-2 lineage B.1.1.7 in Slovakia using a novel, multiplexed RT-qPCR assay. Sci Rep 2021; 11(1):20494.
78. Wang H, Jean S, Eltringham R, et al. Mutation-specific SARS-CoV-2 PCR screen: rapid and accurate detection of variants of concern and the identification of a newly emerging variant with spike L452R mutation. J Clin Microbiol 2021;59(8): e0092621.
79. Wang H, Miller JA, Verghese M, et al. Multiplex SARS-CoV-2 genotyping reverse transcriptase PCR for population-level variant screening and epidemiologic surveillance. J Clin Microbiol 2021;59(8):e0085921.
80. Vandenberg O, Martiny D, Rochas O, et al. Considerations for diagnostic COVID-19 tests. Nat Rev Microbiol 2021;19(3):171–83.
81. In vitro diagnostics EUAs - molecular diagnostic tests for SARS-CoV-2. Available at: https://www.fda.gov/medical-devices/coronavirus-disease-2019-covid-19-emergency-use-authorizations-medical-devices/in-vitro-diagnostics-euas-molecular-diagnostic-tests-sars-cov-2. accessed 6/23/2021.
82. Cyranoski D. Alarming COVID variants show vital role of genomic surveillance. Nature 2021;589(7842):337–8.
83. Smith E, Zhen W, Manji R, et al. Analytical and clinical comparison of three nucleic acid amplification tests for SARS-CoV-2 detection. J Clin Microbiol 2020; 58(9):e01134-20.
84. Zhen W, Manji R, Smith E, et al. Comparison of four molecular in vitro diagnostic assays for the detection of SARS-CoV-2 in nasopharyngeal specimens. J Clin Microbiol 2020;58(8):e00743-20.
85. Craney AR, Velu PD, Satlin MJ, et al. Comparison of two high-throughput reverse transcription-PCR systems for the detection of severe acute respiratory syndrome Coronavirus 2. J Clin Microbiol 2020;58(8):e00890-20.
86. Degli-Angeli E, Dragavon J, Huang ML, et al. Validation and verification of the Abbott Real-Time SARS-CoV-2 assay analytical and clinical performance. J Clin Virol 2020;129:104474.
87. Kogoj R, Kmetic P, Valencak AO, et al. Real-life head-to-head comparison of performance of two high-throughput automated assays for detection of SARS-CoV-2 RNA in nasopharyngeal swabs: the Alinity m SARS-CoV-2 and cobas 6800 SARS-CoV-2 assays. J Mol Diagn 2021;23(8):920–8.

88. Lima A, Healer V, Vendrone E, et al. Validation of a modified CDC assay and performance comparison with the NeuMoDx and DiaSorin(R) automated assays for rapid detection of SARS-CoV-2 in respiratory specimens. J Clin Virol 2020;133: 104688.
89. Mostafa HH, Lamson DM, Uhteg K, et al. Multicenter evaluation of the NeuMoDx SARS-CoV-2 test. J Clin Virol 2020;130:104583.

Approaches to Deployment of Molecular Testing for SARS-CoV-2 in Resource-Limited Settings

Gama Bandawe, PhD[a],*, Moses Chitenje, BSc[b,c],
Joseph Bitiliyu-Bangoh, MSc[d], Elizabeth Kampira, PhD[e]

KEYWORDS

- SARS-CoV-2 • Molecular testing • Laboratory strengthening
- National reference laboratory • Cost reduction

KEY POINTS

- Deployment of molecular testing in resource-limited settings needs to be approached in the broader context of laboratory strengthening.
- Scale-up of molecular testing was built on existing pathogen control programs for human immunodeficiency virus and tuberculosis.
- National reference laboratories have an essential role to play in successful roll out of molecular testing.
- Pooled testing and direct-to-polymerase chain reaction methods have great potential for cost saving and increasing access to molecular testing.

INTRODUCTION

Less than a month after severe acute respiratory syndrome coronavirus-2 (SARS-CoV-2) was described as the causative agent of COVID-19,[1,2] molecular diagnostic assays based on reverse transcriptase qualitative polymerase chain reaction (RT-qPCR) were rapidly developed.[3] In the absence of other sensitive and reliable methods, these assays became the primary method that enabled countries around the globe to identify and the

[a] Biological Sciences Department, Academy of Medical Sciences, Malawi University of Science and Technology, P. O. Box 5196, Limbe, Malawi; [b] International Teaching and Education Centre for Health (ITECH), PO Box 30369, Capital City Lilongwe 3, Plot 13/14, 1st Floor ARWA House, City Center, Lilongwe, Malawi; [c] Public Health Institute of Malawi, Ministry of Health, Lilongwe, Malawi; [d] Ministry of Health, P.O. Box 30377, Lilongwe 3, Malawi; [e] Centres for Disease Control and Prevention, P. O. Box 30016, NICO House, City Centre, Lilongwe 3, Lilongwe, Malawi
* Corresponding author.
E-mail address: gbandawe@must.ac.mw

Clin Lab Med 42 (2022) 283–298
https://doi.org/10.1016/j.cll.2022.02.008
0272-2712/22/© 2022 Elsevier Inc. All rights reserved.

disease, conduct surveillance, and mount a response to the pandemic. Use of this assay as a routine diagnostic tool in many parts of the world was limited, as it is relatively specialized requiring some complex machinery, infrastructure, and training to conduct competently and routinely with high throughput. The World Health Organization (WHO) published testing guidelines,[4–6] which included biosafety level 2 conditions for handling of specimens for molecular testing. Although these requirements pose a challenge even in the most affluent countries, in resource-limited settings they presented an even more significant challenge. Despite this, molecular testing capacity had to be rapidly scaled up to meet the testing needs in every part of the world. Here the authors outline some of the key considerations, partnerships, and activities that were required and draw on several specific examples from Malawi in Southern Africa. Lessons drawn from this experience can be informative for continued laboratory strengthening and preparation for any future outbreaks of novel zoonotic or reemerging pathogens of public health concern.

SYSTEMS STRENGTHENING

Low- and middle-income countries are often those with the highest disease burden, and lack of adequate laboratory capacity presents a further barrier in provision of appropriate diagnosis, care, and treatment of existing diseases and emerging pathogens.[7–9] The establishment of fully equipped testing laboratories that fulfill WHO guidelines required huge investment, expertise, and time, which are limited by the many other competing priorities and requirements of a national COVID-19 response. Laboratory systems in many low- and middle-income countries were already struggling under the weight of a myriad of systemic challenges including lack of laboratory supplies, lack of essential equipment, limited numbers of skilled personnel, lack of educators and training programs, inadequate logistical support, deemphasis of laboratory testing, insufficient monitoring of test quality, decentralization of laboratory facilities, and lack of government standards for laboratory testing.[9] Efforts to scale-up any disease response would need to therefore be conducted using a broader systems strengthening approach that attempts to address many of these issues concurrently.

In the last 2 decades, a significant amount of funding and investment has flowed into strengthening of laboratories[10,11] mainly aligned with specific pathogen control programs especially human immunodeficiency virus (HIV), tuberculosis (TB), and malaria. With HIV control programs, improved laboratory capacity has resulted from the need to provide comprehensive laboratory diagnostic services for monitoring patients on antiretroviral therapy with CD4, chemistry, hematology, testing for HIV-1 drug resistance mutations and testing for opportunistic infections.[12] Importantly, there was also a need for molecular tests for detecting and measuring plasma RNA levels via RT-qPCR for early infant diagnosis and detection of treatment failure or viremic control as part of the treatment cascade.[13] With the TB control programs, the need to provide rapid molecular point-of-care detection as well as detection of rifampicin resistance[14] was essential. Both of these programs proved to be invaluable in providing a meaningful platform that the deployment of molecular testing for SARS-CoV-2 could build on.

The exigency of using existing infrastructure and capacity to pivot onto the COVID response reinforced the need for continued emphasis on integration of laboratory services and capacity to meet a diversity of needs, which we have now learned can evolve rapidly. This integrated laboratory system approach, in contrast to the disease-specific programs, moves toward provision of quality-assured basic laboratory testing through the use of common specimen collection, reporting and diagnostic platforms that can be used across diseases, and disease control programs, and it increases capacity for introducing and using new and more complex technologies.[12]

ROLE OF THE NATIONAL REFERENCE LABORATORY

Globally, national reference laboratories play a central role in the implementation of any disease response and especially the scale-up of diagnostic capacity. In the context of resource-limited settings where capacity may not have existed or needed to be significantly boosted, the importance of this facility is heightened further. National Reference Laboratories are at the pinnacle of diagnostic service provision and play pivotal roles in diagnosis, disease surveillance, and statistical analysis of epidemiologic data. In 2009 the Southern Africa Development Community set out the functions and minimum standards for national reference laboratories that must be achieved and maintained by all its member states. The functions included general diagnostics (specialized testing services especially molecular testing), development and implementation of diagnostic policy, maintaining diagnostic standards, training and skills transfers, servicing and maintenance of equipment, provision of quality management systems, information management, and public health functions. The main public health functions of national reference laboratories that were specified involve coordination of the following: surveillance and epidemic response, training, qualifications and continuing professional education, operational research for health, laboratory health and safety, specimen handling, and transportation.[15]

In Malawi, the Public Health Institute of Malawi (PHIM), under the Malawi Ministry of Health alongside its department of Health Technical Support Services, activated the Public Health Emergency Operations Center to coordinate the national COVID-19 response. Under PHIM, the Public Health Reference Laboratory (PHL) is the coordinating body for the tiered laboratory system that includes national and reference laboratories in the upper tier, central laboratories based in the country's major referral hospitals, and a lower tier of peripheral laboratories in district hospitals and health centers. PHL also coordinates private sector and academic laboratories within the country.

One of the most important roles spearheaded by the PHL was the coordination of multiple partners in the many activities required to successfully capacitate the health system to conduct high-throughput molecular testing and make it as widely available as possible. **Table 1** gives a snapshot of some of the most important activities undertaken and the partners involved. Alongside the Ministry of Health, at least 10 different international organizations and regional partners were involved in supporting the various activities under the thematic areas of equipment, infrastructure, personnel, procurement of reagents and consumables, training, sample transportation, data management, and quality management.

Other key functions of the PHL were decisions on the scale of the diagnostic response, determination and development of guidelines, and validation and approval of which specific tests, reagents, and platforms would be used. This particular issue took on magnified importance for several reasons. The disruptions to global supply chains brought about by lockdowns and international travel bans as well as unprecedented demand for molecular testing supplies and reagents meant that the demand for testing was never going to be matched by the supply. Data from the Association of Supply Chain Management and the American Society for Microbiology showed that worldwide shortages of media, reagents, collection devices, and consumables

Table 1
Summary of some of the activities undertaken to achieve successful roll out of molecular testing services for SARS–CoV-2 in Malawi under 8 thematic areas

Thematic Area	Activities	Partners	Main Outcomes/Highlights
Equipment	Inventory of available platforms	MoH	Updated inventory available at central level
			Identification of 22 high-throughput platforms across the country for molecular testing facilitated planning, procurement, and distribution of supplies
	Servicing and calibration of equipment	MoH CDC Malawi through UMB	Auxiliary equipment with valid calibration certificates. Securing of service contracts
			Ensuring availability of calibrators through implementing partners
	Biosafety cabinets	CDC Malawi through UMB	Functional and fully serviced biosafety cabinets in every testing site
	Procurement of Abbott m2000 platform GeneXpert machines Quant Studio 5	CDC Malawi Thermofisher USAID	Scaled up capacity for molecular testing
Infrastructure	Demarcation/partitioning of laboratories for molecular testing	MoH, CDC Malawi through UMB	All sites partitioned to accommodate separate molecular testing.
personnel	Recruitment of additional laboratory	MoH CDC Malawi through UMB	Additional 150 laboratory personnel recruited. Repurposing of UMB staff to support COVID testing. Uninterrupted service for other molecular assays due to adequate personnel

Procurement of reagents and consumables	Determining needs	MoH CDC Malawi through UMB and I-TECH	Constant supply of reagents Sufficient supply of reagents
	Coordination with development partners	MoH	Ensured collaborative effort and maximum resource allocation Monitoring of reagents and distribution to various testing sites
	Supply chain and logistics	UNICEF/WFP Central Medical Stores Trust CHAI, I-TECH	Ensured delivery of reagents, supplies, and PPE amid global supply chain constraints
Training	Training in sample collection and processing	MoH CDC Malawi through I-TECH CDC Zambia WHO, World Bank	Training of laboratory officers in SARS-CoV-2 testing to scale-up testing capacity Supported initial TOT for PCR testing 25,000 health workers trained in sample collection
Sample transportation	Development of a transportation system	UMB/Riders for Health	Successful transportation of 231,850 samples to molecular laboratories. Transportation from ports of entry and hard to reach areas.
Data management	Production of case-based surveillance form	MoH	Standardization of data
	Development of a national dashboard	I-TECH	Stakeholders are able to access data through the dashboard
	connectivity	EGPAF	Majority (85%) of testing sites are connected to the dash board

(continued on next page)

Table 1
(continued)

Thematic Area	Activities	Partners	Main Outcomes/Highlights
Quality management	Approval of laboratories to perform SARS-CoV-2 PCR testing	MoH-HTSS	15 molecular laboratories and 320 antigen testing sites have been approved
	Validation of different platforms	PHL	Validated 3 molecular platforms and 4 antigen test kits
			All molecular assays in use validated in county against available platforms
	EQA	PHIM supported by UMB	Ensured accurate result generation using annual EQA with score of 94%

Full names of key partners and organisations are given below the table

Abbreviations: CDC, Centers for Disease Control and Prevention; CHAI, Clinton Health Access Initiative; EGPAF, Elizabeth Glazer Paediatric AIDS Foundation; HTSS, Health Technical Support Services; I-TECH, International Training and Education Center for Health; PHL, Public Health Laboratory; MoH, Ministry of Health; UMB, University of Maryland Baltimore; UNICEF, United Nations Children's Fund; USAID, United States Agency for International Development; WFP, World Food Program; WHO, World Health Organization.

significantly affected day-to-day testing for both COVID-19 and other infectious diseases.[16] These shortages were more acute in resource-limited settings, and many countries had to make do with whatever they could get access to. At the same time, there was a flood of newly developed tests reagents and consumables that were yet to be validated that became available on the market. Sensitivity of molecular tests is greatly affected by proper specimen collection, and a myriad of swabs, specimen collection kits, and viral transportation media also became available and were aggressively marketed. In addition to issuing comprehensive guidelines in sample collection, much work had to be put in to validate the performance of and approve which product could be used by health workers and laboratory staff to ensure the quality of molecular diagnostic results.

POLYMERASE CHAIN REACTION PLATFORMS

Molecular diagnostic (PCR) systems for SARS-CoV-2 provide extremely sensitive, specific, and often quantitative detection of the SARS-CoV-2 RNA. However, they are complex, expensive, and slow to deliver. A single RT-PCR test kit may cost more than 100USD, whereas setting up a diagnostic/processing laboratory requires more than 15,000 USD, whereas the analysis time is 4 to 6 hours, and sample-to-result turn-around time is often more than 24 hours.[17,18] A PCR system includes PCR kit, PCR machine, and PCR software, and all RT-PCR systems are different due to differences in kit chemistry, thermal profile, PCR kinetics, and so forth.[19] An additional issue is the fact that different kits are compatible with different machines, and they have specific versions and software. Scale-up of molecular testing needed to account for all of these differences and circumvent issues related to this. Procurement of testing kits and receipt of donations needed to be done based on an up-to-date inventory of the available systems and their compatibility with different machines. Compatibility of different test kits with instruments along with sensitivities, limits of detection, cycle threshold value cut-offs, and the required consumables are detailed by FIND[20] and the Global Fund.[21]

In Malawi, 4 laboratories were initially optimized to perform RT-qPCR using US-CDC ThermoFisher TaqMan and DaanGene protocols on Applied Biosystem 7500 and Abbott m2000sp/m2000rt instruments.[22] The DaanGene kits were part of a donation of 1.5 million laboratory diagnostic test kits and more than 100 tons of infection prevention and control commodities from the Jack Ma and Alibaba Foundations made in March 2020.[23] An initial 20,000 kits were donated to each member state, and for many African countries this was the most widely available kit. The kit is manufactured by the DaAn Gene Co., Ltd. of Sun Yat-sen University, Guangdong, China and is based on one-step RT-PCR technique. It contains an endogenous internal standard detection system, which was used for monitoring the processes of specimen collection, RNA, and PCR amplification, thereby reducing false-negative results. The kit is compatible with ABI PRISM 7500 SDS and LightCycler480 II instruments.

An important consideration is the maintenance of the cold chain when shipping test kits from the manufacturer as well as when distributing the kits to central and peripheral laboratories. In the face if logistical challenges associated with this, kits that have lyophilized components were favored in procurement processes. Kits such as the TIB Molbiol (Berlin GmbH/Roche Diagnostics) were preferred because the product is dried and is stored at 4°C to 25°C enabling shipping without temperature control. Although some challenges persist with instability of enzymes once reconstituted, advances in development of room-temperature–storable PCR mixes for SARS-CoV-2 detection[24] offer some promise in this regard and would be a welcome boost to molecular testing in resource-limited settings.

Abbott Platform

The Abbott RealTime HIV-1 Qualitative test (Abbott Diagnostics, Inc., Chicago Illinois, USA) is an RT-PCR–based assay for the qualitative detection of HIV type 1 (HIV-1) nucleic acids from human plasma and dried blood spots. The RealTime HIV-1 Qualitative test is intended to be used as an aid in the diagnosis of HIV-1 infection in pediatric and adult subjects. It is designed to be run on the Abbott RealTime m2000rt amplification system or the fully automated m24 system. The RealTime HIV-1 is included in a Global Fund framework agreement as part of an expanded assay menu—together with HIV early infant diagnosis, mycobacterium tuberculosis (MTB), hepatitis B virus, hepatitis C virus, human papillomavirus, and Chlamydia trachomatis/Neisseria gonorrhoeae—at the same low access price. Abbott offers scale-up planning as well as assistance with scale-up, including training and performance monitoring based on country needs.[25] For this reason, it has become a key component in the global HIV program as well as laboratory systems strengthening programs and thus has a presence in most countries supported by PEPFAR and Global Fund programs.

The FDA-approved Abbott's RealTime SARS-CoV-2 assay is a dual-target RT-PCR assay for the quantitative recognition of RdRp and N genes. It uses an unrelated RNA sequence as an internal control (IC) to validate the PCR and detects the RdRp, N, and IC target sequences via specific fluorescent-labeled probes. Different fluorophores are used for SARS-CoV-2–specific and IC-specific probes to allow simultaneous detection of these targets[26]; this became one of the first tests that was deployed in Malawi and was used in the detection of the first case in the country in March 2020 at the National reference laboratory and College of Medicine and the Malawi Liverpool Wellcome Trust laboratories. By April 2020, additional molecular laboratories were activated to extend testing to additional districts using the Abbott test kit and m2000sp/m2000rt instruments (**Fig. 1**A).[22]

GeneXpert

GeneXpert (Cepheid, Inc., Sunnyvale, CA) is a cartridge-based PCR machine that is used to diagnose TB and detect rifampicin resistance. Following its endorsement of Xpert MTB/RIF by the WHO in 2010, its implementation across the globe has

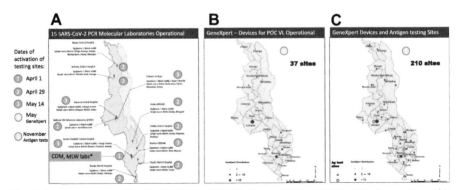

Fig. 1. Map of testing sites for SARS-CoV-2 in Malawi. (*A*) The 15 RT-qPCR sites activated in the first 2 months from April 2020 to May 2020. (*B*) The activation of GeneXpert sites (37) in all districts of the country. (*C*) The rapid antigen testing sites activated in November of 2020 (210 sites).

revolutionized management of TB and has become the bedrock of many national TB control programs.[27] The cartridge-based modular diagnostic tool has enabled the rapid diagnosis of critically ill cases and assessment of suspected patients, allowing for a specific epidemiologic management. The biggest advantage has been the transfer diagnostics to point-of-care scenarios including smaller peripheral laboratories. Public health experts in low- and middle-income countries were quick to see its potential in expanding testing capacity and called for production of cartridges for SARS-CoV-2 detection.[28] The Xpert Xpress SARS-CoV-2 cartridge was granted emergency use authorization in March 2020.

In Malawi there was at least one GeneXpert platform in each of the country's 26 districts, and by the May of 2020 SARS-CoV-2 testing on this platform was available in each district (**Fig. 1**B). By August 2020 there were 37 sites across the country.[29] The GeneXpert platform became the most important tool enabling the establishment of near point-of-care molecular testing capacity at ports of entry where local laboratories had limited capacity but the need for accurate testing with rapid turn-around time was greatest.

IMPACT ON TUBERCULOSIS AND HUMAN IMMUNODEFICIENCY VIRUS CONTROL PROGRAMS

The negative impact of COVID-19 on health care systems in general as well as on pathogen control programs was certainly expected and anticipated.[30] The lockdowns and health facility closures seen early in the pandemic were especially damaging to mass vaccination campaigns for measles, polio, and meningitis and left millions of children at increased risk.[31] The shift in focus resulted in massive redeployment of human and financial resources, delays, and disruptions in supply chains of essential medicines and equipment. The most direct impact of the scale-up in molecular testing for SARS-CoV-2 was in the shifting of testing platforms and skilled personnel from HIV and TB control programs.[32] This process had to be managed in a circumspect manner to mitigate any negative impacts, and policy makers and planners were acutely aware of this. In many facilities, machines were shared and rotated between testing for HIV/TB and testing for SARS-CoV-2, and this situation continues today. Some countries' TB programs saw up to a 70% reduction in new TB case detection[31] but this was mainly attributed to factors such as decreased patient flows.[33] For HIV programs despite some countries experiencing decreases of greater than 50% in HIV testing and greater than 10% increase in deaths from opportunistic infections,[34] in PEPFAR-supported countries there was only a 7% drop in provision of viral load testing services.[32] In several countries many HIV testing services experienced minimal disruption, and viral load testing coverage levels were restored to prepandemic levels or better due to swift measures taken by health officials. In Malawi, routine viral load testing was suspended from March to June of 2020 but quickly saw rebounds to prepandemic levels once the suspension was lifted. Some specific and impactful government measures included providing guidance on continuing essential services, increasing the number of viral load specimen pick-ups at testing facilities, expanding collection of dried blood spot specimens (which can be stored and transported without refrigeration) relative to plasma specimens, and integrating viral load testing with antiretroviral therapy distribution[32] and implementation of remote viral load supervision using mobile phones.[35]

TRANSITION TO ANTIGEN TESTS AND USE CASES FOR MOLECULAR TESTS

The development of and transition to rapid antigen tests provided relief to strained central and peripheral testing sites relying on RT-qPCR and enabled significant decentralization and scale-up of testing. The public health impact was massive, as most of the individuals suspecting COVID-19 infection go first to the local clinics where RT-qPCR was most often not available. In Malawi the use of rapid antigen testing resulted in an increase of testing sites from 37 (with conventional PCR and GeneXpert) to 210 across the country (**Fig. 1C**). Numerous studies have been conducted on the performance of these tests relative to PCR-based tests and have consistently found reductions in sensitivity particularly in asymptomatic subjects.[36–38] This is considered an acceptable trade-off for the high number of tests being conducted and for the fact that patients who are the most infectious are more likely to test positive. The huge reduction in turn-around time and the ability to conduct more frequent and repeated test use are also seen a compensating for the loss in sensitivity.[38,39]

In spite of all the foregoing, several use cases remain for PCR-based testing. Most countries around the world have a requirement for an RT-qPCR negative result both for entry and exit, and airlines will not allow passengers to board without it.[40] Many countries are loosening guidelines for isolation in an attempt to reduce the amount of economic disruption of COVID infections[41,42] and do not require a negative PCR test for discharge, opting rather for a negative antigen test. In Malawi, the guidelines do not rely on PCR-based or antigen tests for discharge[43] but require a minimum of 10 days in isolation, 3 of which have to be symptom free; this is mainly because it is known that some individuals may continue to test positive for months[44] and providing a second antigen test may prove difficult even with the current availability of antigen testing.

Another use of PCR testing is in environmental monitoring for SARS-CoV-2. Because of extended shedding and excretion of SARS-CoV-2 RNA in fecal matter, water-based epidemiology is now recognized as a potentially important means of surveillance of SARS-CoV-2 transmission and real-time trend monitoring.[45] The methodologies used are based on RT-qPCR analysis of sewage or waste water.[46] This method of surveillance can predict surges in cases with a lead time of up to 2 weeks, and in densely populated urban areas in developing countries this approach could be superior to clinical surveillance for real-time monitoring of disease trends.[45] However, much methodological development still needs to take place in this area before it can be deployed on a routine basis especially in resource limited settings. Unlike clinical samples, detection of viruses in environmental samples is challenging due to the low-concentration virus present, and this makes it necessary to concentrate the sample, and the presence of fecal and suspended solids and chemicals induced by domestic usage, urban and rural runoffs, and industrial activities makes amplification difficult.[46,47]

APPROACHES TO COST REDUCTION

Several approaches have been considered in an effort to reduce costs of molecular testing and thereby widen access to testing in resource-limited settings. Pooling of samples, direct-to-PCR testing procedures, usage of simpler sampling methods such as saliva, and technologies such as isothermal PCR reactions and colorimetric PCR-based viral detection methodologies have all been proposed.[48–51] The last 2 approaches are promising and are reviewed elsewhere in this edition. The former 2 however seem to offer rapid and immediate relief on already stretched resources.

Pooled Testing

Pooling involves pipetting equal amounts of multiple samples into one tube, enabling one to screen multiple patients at a go in batches that can then be retested to identify positive samples within each batch. This sort of sample pooling strategy has routinely been used for detection of the HIV and hepatitis B and C viruses in blood bank donor screening in many countries and dating back many years.[52] By some estimates using a pooling strategy for SARS-CoV-2 detection can reduce cost by 69% and requires 10-fold fewer tests.[53] Pools of up to 32 samples can successfully be used with a 10% false-negative rate.[54] However, a balance must be struck between increasing the group size and retaining test sensitivity, as sample dilution increases the likelihood of false-negative test results for individuals with low viral load at the time of the testing.[55] Similarly, minimizing the number of tests to reduce costs must be balanced against minimizing the time that testing takes, as the process is quite labor intensive.[56] Realistically, smaller batches of 10 or fewer give an acceptable false-negative rate samples, and high intra- and interassay variability is observed especially where low viral load samples are present.[53,57] In addition, the pooling is only cost-effective when prevalence is low[57,58] and for screening natural groupings with correlated risks of infection amenable to repeated mass testing such as workplaces, prisons, schools, and other institutions. None the less, this strategy has been used with varying degrees of success in Ghana,[56] Uganda,[59] Rwanda, and South Africa.[58]

Simplified Extraction and Straight to Polymerase Chain Reaction Methods

In currently used RT-qPCR methods RNA extraction constitutes a major bottleneck that requires a significant quantity of consumable plastics and chemical reagents to complete.[60] Few laboratories' resource-limited settings have automated extraction robots, and RNA extraction kits are among those reagents affected by increased demand and global supply chain challenges. One solution is to bypass the RNA extraction step, which would result in reduction of analysis time, savings in reagents and consumables, reductions in waste, and possibly expand the number of nonspecialized laboratories able to perform COVID-19 diagnosis.[61–63] Studies have shown good sensitivity with extraction-free PCR assays, especially for high viral loads[62] and others have shown that the extraction step can be bypassed if samples are stored in universal transport medium or molecular grade water but not when stored in saline or Hanks medium.[61] One study conducted in Malawi using a direct-to-PCR methodology was able to achieve significant savings in cost and processing time by using a 30-second mechanical homogenization step versus an hour-long reagent heavy extraction procedure.[63] This approach is particularly promising and has potential to be scaled up to all molecular laboratories.

CONCLUDING REMARKS AND FUTURE DIRECTIONS

Significant challenges have had to be surmounted in the deployment of molecular testing for SARS-CoV-2 in resource-limited setting but it has played an essential role in the global response to COVID-19. Continued progress in strengthening of laboratory systems, integration, and development of increased technical and human capacity will ensure that gains made in this area are not lost and will safeguard the ability of health care systems and medical laboratory scientists to be better prepared and equipped for future pandemics. There is also a need to intensify research into development of platforms, and more cost-saving methodologies that are better suited for lower- and middle-income countries are fully harnessed to effectively address gaps and challenges that remain. In particular, field trials and implementation research coupled with robust qualitative studies that can lead to scale-up of some of these approaches are emphasized. There is also a role for increased partnerships and technology transfer to enable building of local manufacturing capacity to allow more countries to develop their own capacity to supply their health sectors with much needed reagents and supplies for molecular diagnostics. Some encouraging examples of this have been illustrated in countries such as South Africa,[64] Senegal, and Brazil where agencies such as FIND and UNITAID have partnered with local forms to achieve this in antigen testing.[65] Similar endeavors related to molecular testing would be a welcome development.

CLINICS CARE POINTS

- Molecular testing for SARS-CoV-2 in many settings is dependent on GeneXpert and Abbott platforms.
- Scale up of testing has pargely been well handled to minimise the impact on HIV and TB control programs.
- Introduction of rapid antibody testing has enabled increases in testing capacity and reach and it has simutlaneously releived pressure on infrastructure, equipment and personnel.

DISCLOSURE

Gama Bandawe is funded by the Malawi University of Science and Technology. The other authors have nothing to disclose.

REFERENCES

1. Zhou P, Yang X-L, Wang X-G, et al. A pneumonia outbreak associated with a new coronavirus of probable bat origin. Nature 2020;579(7798):270–3.
2. Gorbalenya AE, Baker SC, Baric RS, et al. The species Severe acute respiratory syndrome-related coronavirus: classifying 2019-nCoV and naming it SARS-CoV-2. Nat Microbiol 2020;5(4):536–44.
3. Chan JF-W, Yip CC-Y, To KK-W, et al. Improved molecular diagnosis of COVID-19 by the novel, highly sensitive and specific COVID-19-RdRp/Hel real-time reverse Transcription-PCR assay validated in Vitro and with clinical specimens. J Clin Microbiol 2020;58(5). https://doi.org/10.1128/JCM.00310-20.
4. Cao W, Liu X, Bai T, et al. High-dose intravenous immunoglobulin as a therapeutic option for deteriorating patients with Coronavirus Disease 2019. Open Forum Infect Dis 2020;48:1–6.
5. World Health Organization. Laboratory testing for coronavirus disease 2019 (COVID-19) in suspected human cases, WHO. Interim Guidance 2020.
6. World health Organization. Laboratory testing strategy recommendations for COVID-19. World heal organ. 2020. Available at: https://apps.who.int/iris/bitstream/handle/10665/331509/WHO-COVID-19-lab_testing-2020.1-eng.pdf.
7. Vitoria M, Granich R, Gilks CF, et al. The global fight against HIV/AIDS, tuberculosis, and Malaria: current Status and future Perspectives. Am J Clin Pathol 2009;131(6):844–8.
8. Birx D, de Souza M, Nkengasong JN. Laboratory challenges in the scaling up of HIV, TB, and Malaria programs: the Interaction of health and laboratory systems, clinical research, and service delivery. Am J Clin Pathol 2009;131(6):849–51.
9. Petti CA, Polage CR, Quinn TC, et al. Laboratory medicine in Africa: a barrier to effective health care. Clin Infect Dis 2006;42(3):377–82.

10. Ravishankar N, Gubbins P, Cooley RJ, et al. Financing of global health: tracking development assistance for health from 1990 to 2007. Lancet 2009;373(9681): 2113–24.

11. Yu D, Souteyrand Y, Banda MA, et al. Investment in HIV/AIDS programs: Does it help strengthen health systems in developing countries? Glob Health 2008;4(1): 8. https://doi.org/10.1186/1744-8603-4-8.

12. Parsons LM, Somoskovi A, Lee E, et al. Global health: integrating national laboratory health systems and services in resource-limited settings. Afr J Lab Med 2011;1(1):1–5.

13. UNAIDS. Fast-Track Ending the AIDS Pandemic by 2030.; 2014.

14. Steingart KR, Schiller I, Horne DJ, et al. Xpert® MTB/RIF assay for pulmonary tuberculosis and rifampicin resistance in adults. Cochrane Database Syst Rev 2014;1. https://doi.org/10.1002/14651858.CD009593.pub3.

15. SADC. Functions and Minimum Standards for National Reference Laboratories in the SADC Region. Published online 2009.

16. American Society for Microbiology. Supply shortages impacting COVID-19 and non-COVID testing Title. 2021. Available at: https://asm.org/Articles/2020/September/Clinical-Microbiology-Supply-Shortage-Collecti-1. Accessed January 10, 2022.

17. Ramdas K, Darzi A, Jain S. 'Test, re-test, re-test': using inaccurate tests to greatly increase the accuracy of COVID-19 testing. Nat Med 2020;26(6):810–1.

18. Sheridan C. Fast, portable tests come online to curb coronavirus pandemic. Nat Biotechnol 2020;38(5):515–8.

19. Das P, Mondal S, Pal S, et al. COVID diagnostics by molecular methods : a systematic review of nucleic acid based testing systems. Indian J Med Microbiol 2020;39(3):271–8.

20. Find. Find EVALUATION UPDATE: SARS-COV-2 molecular diagnostics. 2022. Available at: https://www.finddx.org/covid-19/sarscov2-eval-molecular/.

21. Global Fund. List of SARS-CoV-2 Diagnostic test kits and equipments eligible for procurement according to Board Decision on Additional Support for Country Responses to COVID-19 (GF/B42/EDP11) SARS-CoV-2 Nucleic Acid Amplification Technologies (only sequencing e 2022;19:1–74.

22. Ministry of Health of Malawi. MALAWI SARS-COV-2 DIAGNOSIS NATIONAL LABORATORY GUIDELINE, Ministry of Health Malawi, Manual, 1, 2020.

23. Africa CDC. Jack Ma and Alibaba Foundations donate COVID-19 medical equipment to African union member states. 2020. Available at: https://africacdc.org/news-item/jack-ma-and-alibaba-foundations-donate-covid-19-medical-equipment-to-african-union-member-states/. Accessed January 15, 2022.

24. Xu J, Wang J, Zhong Z, Su X, Yang K, Chen Z. Room-temperature-storable PCR mixes for SARS-CoV-2 detection. *Clinical Biochemistry* (84) 73-78;2020.

25. Mazzola LT, Perez-Casas C. HIV/AIDS Diagnostics Technology Landscape. *UNITAID*. 5th edition. Report; 2015.

26. Abbott. Abbott RealTime SARS-C0V-2 assay. 2021. Available at: https://www.molecular.abbott/int/en/products/infectious-disease/RealTime-SARS-CoV-2-Assay. Accessed February 22, 2022.

27. Brown S, Leavy JE, Jancey J. Implementation of GeneXpert for TB testing in low- and middle-income countries: a systematic review. Glob Heal Sci Pract 2021; 9(3):698. https://doi.org/10.9745/GHSP-D-21-00121. LP - 710.

28. Oladimeji O, Atiba BP, Adeyinka DA. Leveraging polymerase chain reaction technique (GeneXpert) to upscaling testing capacity for SARS-CoV-2 (COVID-19) in

Nigeria: a game changer. Pan Afr Med J 2020;35(Supp 2):8–9. https://doi.org/10.11604/pamj.2020.35.2.22693.

29. Public Health Institute of Malawi. COVID-19 Daily situation report - 30th. 2020;(August):1-8.

30. Togun T, Kampmann B, Stoker NG, et al. Anticipating the impact of the COVID-19 pandemic on TB patients and TB control programmes. Ann Clin Microbiol Antimicrob 2020;19(1):21.

31. Roberts L. How COVID hurt the fight against other dangerous diseases. Nature 2021;592(7855):502–4.

32. Lecher SL, Naluguza M, Mwangi C, et al. Notes from the field: impact of the COVID-19 response on scale-up of HIV viral load testing — PEPFAR-supported countries, January–June 2020. MMWR Morb Mortal Wkly Rep 2021;70(21):794–5.

33. Chopra KK, Matta S, Arora VK. Impact of second wave of Covid-19 on tuberculosis control. Indian J Tuberc 2021;68(3):311–2.

34. Medina N, Alastruey-Izquierdo A, Bonilla O, et al. Impact of the COVID-19 pandemic on HIV care in Guatemala. Int J Infect Dis IJID Off Publ Int Soc Infect Dis 2021;108:422–7.

35. Masiano S, Dunga S, Tembo T, et al. Implementing remote supervision to improve HIV service delivery in rural Malawi. J Glob Heal Rep 2020;(VI):1–11.

36. Muthamia E, Mungai S, Mungai M, et al. Assessment of performance and implementation characteristics of rapid point of care sars-cov-2 antigen testing in kenya. medRxiv 2021. https://doi.org/10.1101/2021.06.03.21258290.

37. Amer RM, Samir M, Gaber OA, et al. Diagnostic performance of rapid antigen test for COVID-19 and the effect of viral load, sampling time, subject's clinical and laboratory parameters on test accuracy. J Infect Public Health 2021;14(10):1446–53.

38. American Society for Microbiology. HomeArticlesReal-world performance of COVID-19 rapid antigen tests real-world performance of COVID-19 rapid antigen tests. 2021. Available at: https://asm.org/Articles/2021/December/Real-World-Performance-of-COVID-19-Rapid-Antigen-T. Accessed January 21, 1022.

39. Kahanec M, Lafférs L, Schmidpeter B. The impact of repeated mass antigen testing for COVID-19 on the prevalence of the disease. J Popul Econ 2021;34(4):1105–40.

40. Travelbans.org. TRAVEL BAN, NEW RULES AND UNEXPECTED FLYING RESTRICTIONS: WHAT will TOURISM be like after CORONAVIRUS?. 2022. Available at: https://travelbans.org/. Accessed February 12, 2022.

41. Limb M. Covid-19: Self-isolation after infection cut to seven days in England. BMJ 2021;375:n3137. https://doi.org/10.1136/bmj.n3137.

42. CDC. CDC Updates and Shortens Recommended isolation and Quarantine Period for general population. 2021. Available at: https://www.cdc.gov/media/releases/2021/s1227-isolation-quarantine-guidance.html. Accessed February 1, 2022.

43. Ministry of Health of Malawi. Covid - 19 Case Management Manual, *Ministry of Health*, Manual; september 2020.

44. Henderson DK, Weber DJ, Babcock H, et al. The perplexing problem of persistently PCR-positive personnel. Infect Control Hosp Epidemiol 2021;42(2):203–4.

45. Kumar M, Joshi M, Kumar A, et al. Unravelling the early warning capability of wastewater surveillance for COVID-19 : a temporal study on SARS-CoV-2 RNA detection and need for the escalation. Environ Res 2021;196(December 2020):110946. https://doi.org/10.1016/j.envres.2021.110946.

46. Hamouda M, Mustafa F, Maraqa M, et al. Science of the Total Environment Wastewater surveillance for SARS-CoV-2 : lessons learnt from recent studies to de fi ne future applications. Sci Total Environ 2021;759:143493.

47. Haramoto E, Kitajima M, Hata A, et al. A review on recent progress in the detection methods and prevalence of human enteric viruses in water. Water Res 2018; 135:168–86.

48. Bokelmann L, Nickel O, Maricic T, et al. Point-of-care bulk testing for SARS-CoV-2 by combining hybridization capture with improved colorimetric LAMP. Nat Commun 2021;12(1):1–8.

49. Garcia-Venzor A, Rueda-Zarazua B, Marquez-Garcia E, et al. SARS-CoV-2 direct detection without RNA isolation with Loop-Mediated isothermal amplification (LAMP) and CRISPR-Cas12. Front Med 2021;8(February):1–9. https://doi.org/ 10.3389/fmed.2021.627679.

50. Morehouse ZP, Proctor CM, Ryan GL, et al. A novel two-step, direct-to-PCR method for virus detection off swabs using human coronavirus 229E. Virol J 2020;17(1):129.

51. Pijuan-galito S, Tarantini FS, Tomlin H, et al. Saliva for COVID-19 testing : Simple but Useless or an Undervalued resource 2021;1(July):1–6.

52. Van TT, Miller J, Warshauer DM, et al. Pooling nasopharyngeal/throat swab specimens to increase testing capacity for influenza viruses by PCR. J Clin Microbiol 2012;50(3):891–6.

53. Mahmoud SA, Ibrahim E, Thakre B, et al. Evaluation of pooling of samples for testing SARS-CoV- 2 for mass screening of COVID-. *BMC Infect Dis* Published Online 2021;1–9.

54. Yelin I, Aharony N, Tamar ES, et al. Evaluation of COVID-19 RT-qPCR test in Multi sample Pools. Clin Infect Dis 2020;71(16):2073–8.

55. Arevalo-Rodriguez I, Buitrago-Garcia D, Simancas-Racines D, et al. False-negative results of initial RT-PCR assays for COVID-19: a systematic review. PLoS One 2020;15(12):e0242958.

56. Asante IA, Adusei-poku M, Bonney HK, et al. Molecular diagnosis for the novel coronavirus SARS-CoV-2 : lessons learnt from the Ghana experience. Ghana Med J 2020;54(4).

57. Nianogo RA, Emeruwa IO, Gounder P, et al. Optimal uses of pooled testing for COVID-19 incorporating imperfect test performance and pool dilution effect: an application to congregate settings in Los Angeles County. J Med Virol 2021; 93(9):5396–404.

58. Mutesa L, Ndishimye P, Butera Y, et al. A pooled testing strategy for identifying SARS-CoV-2 at low prevalence. Nature 2021;589(January). https://doi.org/10. 1038/s41586-020-2885-5.

59. Bogere N, Bongomin F, Katende A, et al. Performance and cost-effectiveness of a pooled testing strategy for SARS-CoV-2 using real-time polymerase chain reaction in Uganda. Int J Infect Dis 2021;113:355–8.

60. Tang Y, Schmitz JE, Persing DH, et al. Laboratory diagnosis of COVID-19: current issues and challenges. Am J Clin Microbiol 2020;(May).

61. Merindol N, Pépin G, Marchand C, et al. SARS-CoV-2 detection by direct rRT-PCR without RNA extraction. J Clin Virol 2020;128(May):104423.

62. Visseaux B, Collin G, Houhou-fidouh N, et al. Evaluation of three extraction-free SARS-CoV-2 RT-PCR assays : a feasible alternative approach with low technical requirements. J Virol Methods 2021;291(November 2020):8–11.

63. Morehouse ZP, Samikwa L, Proctor CM, et al. Validation of a direct-to-PCR COVID-19 detection protocol utilizing mechanical homogenization: a model for

reducing resources needed for accurate testing. PLoS One 2021;16(8 August):1–9.

64. South African Government. SAHPRA approves affordable, locally developed Coronavirus COVID-19 antigen test. 2021. Available at: https://www.gov.za/speeches/sahpra-approves-affordable-locally-developed-coronavirus-covid-19-antigen-test-8-dec-2021.

65. Reuters. Global agencies sign tech transfer deals to boost COVID testing in Africa, Latam. 2021. Available at: https://www.reuters.com/business/healthcare-pharmaceuticals/emb-tech-transfers-boost-antigen-testing-africa-latin-america-2021-07-15/. Accessed December 12, 2021.

Novel Assays for Molecular Detection of Severe Acute Respiratory Syndrome Coronavirus 2

Kyle G. Rodino, PhD, D(ABMM)[a,b], Kenneth P. Smith, PhD, D(ABMM)[c,d], Matthew A. Pettengill, PhD, D(ABMM)[e,*]

KEYWORDS

- SARS-CoV-2 • COVID-19 • Molecular • Variant • Next-generation sequencing
- CRISPR-Cas • Microfluidics

KEY POINTS

- The severe acute respiratory syndrome coronavirus 2 (SARS-CoV-2)/COVID-19 pandemic has placed considerable strain on diagnostic laboratories and driven considerable innovation in viral diagnostic assays.
- Multiple novel technologies, or novel adaptations of existing assays, have been developed that may contribute to diagnostic testing for COVID-19 and eventually other infectious diseases as well.
- Novel approaches to providing at-home or point-of-care diagnostic testing for infectious diseases may improve patient care and public health efforts.

INTRODUCTION

From the onset of the severe acute respiratory syndrome coronavirus 2 (SARS-CoV-2)/COVID-19 pandemic, there has been a major emphasis on molecular laboratory tests for the virus. Shortages in various testing supplies, the desire to increase testing capacity, and a push to make point-of-care or home-based testing available have

All authors contributed equally.
[a] Department of Pathology and Laboratory Medicine, Perelman School of Medicine, University of Pennsylvania, 3400 Spruce Street, 4th Floor Gates Building, Philadelphia, PA 19104, USA; [b] Clinical Microbiology Laboratory, Hospital of the University of Pennsylvania, Philadelphia, PA, USA; [c] Perelman School of Medicine, University of Pennsylvania, Philadelphia, PA, USA; [d] Infectious Disease Diagnostics Laboratory, Children's Hospital of Philadelphia, Main Building 5NW91, 3401 Civic Center Boulevard, Philadelphia, PA 19104, USA; [e] Department of Pathology, Anatomy, and Cell Biology, Thomas Jefferson University, 117 South 11th Street, Pavilion Building, Suite 207, Philadelphia, PA 19107-4998, USA
* Corresponding author.
E-mail address: matthew.pettengill@jefferson.edu
Twitter: @KGRodinoPhD (K.G.R.)

Clin Lab Med 42 (2022) 299–307
https://doi.org/10.1016/j.cll.2022.02.004
0272-2712/22/© 2022 Elsevier Inc. All rights reserved.
labmed.theclinics.com

fostered considerable innovation for SARS-CoV-2 molecular diagnostics, advancements likely to be applicable to other diagnostic uses. The authors attempt to cover some of the most compelling novel types of molecular assays or novel approaches in adapting established molecular methodologies for SARS-CoV-2 detection or characterization.

EFFICIENCY ENHANCING ADAPTATIONS FOR MOLECULAR TESTING

The COVID-19 pandemic led to unprecedented demand for laboratory testing that far outpaced existing capacity. Shortages of supplies and labor exacerbated the problem, resulting in the need for improved efficiency of existing SARS-CoV-2 diagnostics, including specimen pooling and process enhancements. Novel diagnostic methodologies that increase efficiency or speed of testing are discussed elsewhere.

The simplest way to increase testing efficiency is to pool multiple patient specimens in a single reverse transcription–polymerase chain reaction (RT-PCR) reaction. If a pool tests negative, all patients are therefore negative. If the pool tests positive, all patient specimens that comprise that pool must be tested individually to identify the positive patients. However, pooling may reduce sensitivity owing to sample dilution of weakly positive specimens.[1] It is also impractical to implement in high (>10%) prevalence settings where specimen pools are more likely to be positive, necessitating extensive retesting of individual patients.[2] However, as SARS-CoV-2 prevalence decreases, specimen pooling may become an attractive option.

Efficiency can also be enhanced by implementing changes in the typical RT-PCR testing workflow. One of the most significant rate-limiting steps in RT-PCR is the extraction step. This step purifies nucleic acids from the milieu of patient cells and proteins present in primary specimens and reduces inhibitory substances. However, swabs in viral transport media (VTM) are a relatively simple sample matrix, and potential inhibition can easily be assessed by monitoring internal controls, suggesting extraction may not be necessary. As such, laboratories have developed "extraction-free" methods that rely on heat to inactivate virus and lyse cells but lack a traditional nucleic acid purification step. These methodologies are easy to implement and have been demonstrated to be faster than conventional methods while maintaining similar performance characteristics.[3,4]

VARIANT TARGETING POLYMERASE CHAIN REACTION

Viral replication is error prone, leading to mutations in the viral genome.[5] When these mutations confer a selective advantage, genomic variants can emerge and become dominant. From the beginning of the pandemic, variants with mutations deviating from the initial SARS-CoV-2 genomic sequence have be recognized and sorted into a variety of lineage classifications. Beyond these viral phylogenetic relationships, many health organizations have adapted variant classifications based on public health impact, with the Centers for Disease Control and Prevention (CDC) classifying SARS-CoV-2 variants into 3 groups: "variant of interest," "variant of concern," and "variant of high consequence." Each level of classification denotes more significant changes in overall prevalence, viral transmissibility, disease severity, antiviral resistance, and/or vaccine evasion. As such, detection of variants is of epidemiologic, and in some cases clinical, interest.

SARS-CoV-2 variants are first identified by genetic sequencing (often next-generation sequencing [NGS], reviewed elsewhere in this issue). However, sequencing methodologies are time consuming, expensive, and difficult to deploy at large scale as a routine diagnostic. As such, most SARS-CoV-2 tests are performed by other methods, with RT-PCR remaining the gold standard. RT-PCR tests rely on primers and probes that hybridize to known sequences within the viral genome. Therefore, these assays detect sequences for which they were designed with high sensitivity and specificity. However, when faced with a variant containing changes in the assay's genetic target, the virus may evade detection.[6] Furthermore, variants with no changes in the assay's target will be indistinguishable from any other positive result.

In some cases, knowledge of these limitations can be leveraged to identify variants. For example, the assay used in the United Kingdom's national SARS-CoV-2 testing system contains targets for the nucleocapsid gene (N), the spike gene (S), a gene of unknown function (ORFab). In November 2020, a cluster of cases in Kent, England was identified in which the N and ORFab targets yielded positive results, but the S gene was consistently negative (https://assets.publishing.service.gov.uk/government/uploads/system/uploads/attachment_data/file/959360/Variant_of_Concern_VOC_202012_01_Technical_Briefing_3.pdf).

Failure of one or more gene targets in an RT-PCR assay is referred to as gene dropout. This specific pattern of gene dropout was widely recognized and given the name S gene target failure (SGTF). Further investigation of this phenomenon led to the identification of the Alpha SARS-CoV-2 variant (also known as B.1.1.7), which contains a 6-nucleotide deletion within the probe binding site, precluding detection of the S gene. Since this discovery, other assays, including commercially available assays, have used SGTF as a proxy for the Alpha strain.[7] Although positive predictive value of SGTF is good in high-prevalence settings, the Alpha variant's nucleotide deletion also occurs in other variants (notably the Beta variant, also known as B.1.351). Detection of SGTF regained value with the emergence of Omicron, which shared the same deletion in the spike coding region with Alpha. Conveniently, the preceding Delta variant did not contain the same deletion, making SGTF a reliable proxy for classification as Omicron (BA.1).[8,9] This lack of specificity highlights an important limitation of using gene dropout as a detection method and suggests need for variant targeting PCR tests. In addition, relevant to this type of assay generally, the limit of detection (LoD) of the assay can create a "false-dropout" when a particular gene is not detected owing to low positive.

RT-PCR tests can be adapted for variant detection by incorporating variant-specific probes to existing assays. Typically, these would be multiplexed in the same reaction to allow detection of the widest possible number of variants.[10] However, multiplex assays suffer from the same limitations as single-plex assays in that genetic targets must be known in advance. Shifting variant makeup can render a panel with limited mutation targets obsolete or lose specificity if multiple lineages emerge with overlapping mutation combinations, which can be particularly challenging in the clinical laboratory given the significant time and financial investment needed for assay validation. Therefore, unbiased methods, such as genetic sequencing, will likely remain major methods of variant detection.

REVERSE TRANSCRIPTION–POLYMERASE CHAIN REACTION ASSAYS TARGETING REPLICATION INTERMEDIATES

Current CDC guidelines suggest discontinuation of SARS-CoV-2 isolation precautions by a time and symptom-based strategy. Although this policy, based on generalized viral kinetics and disease timeline, may be sufficient when applied broadly, data suggest prolonged disease and extended infectivity in severely immunocompromised populations.[11] Concerns surrounding the duration of infectivity and shedding of viable

SARS-CoV-2 have led to an interest in test-based strategies to determine the transmission potential. Drivers of this approach include informing decisions related to discontinuation of isolation precautions, admission to COVID-19-free units, and transfers to/from facilities, among others. Lacking a definitive test for infectiousness, several methods have been suggested as surrogates of infectivity, each with their own set of challenges.[12] These include repurposing of the cycle threshold (Ct) value obtained from diagnostic RT-PCR assays, which can further complicate interpretation given the qualitative nature of the assays, numerous sources of variability, and the inability to distinguish between live, replicating virus versus residual shedding of genetic material. Although traditional viral culture could serve to detect potentially infectious virus, biosafety considerations, lack of general availability, turnaround time, and questions around sensitivity make this an impractical and reliable option for transmission risk assessment. In an attempt to address these challenges, RT-PCR assays targeting SARS-CoV-2 replication intermediates have been designed. For SARS-CoV-2, a positive-sense, single-stranded RNA (ssRNA) virus, these intermediates, including negative-sense RNA and subgenomic RNAs (sgRNAs), are formed in the host cell as the virus replicates. Theoretically, replication intermediates are only present with viable, actively replicating virus and absent in cases of residual shedding of nonviable genomic RNA in the postinfectious phase.

sgRNAs, fractions of the genome that lead to the production of many viral proteins, have been suggested as diagnostics indicators for active viral replication and presumably productive, transmissible infection. This method, using a leader-specific primer, has been described by Wolfel and colleagues,[13] with sgRNAs sequenced and visualized on agarose gel. Several studies have used this method to assess active replication of SARS-CoV-2.[14–18] However, the presence of sgRNAs as indicators of active replication has been questioned. Other studies have found prolonged detection of sgRNAs, hypothesizing that the membrane-bound nature of SARS-CoV-2 replication provides protection against degradation of these genomic fragments.[19,20] Hogan and colleagues[21] developed and validated a negative-sense RNA RT-PCR assay, independently amplifying positive- and negative-sense RNA of the SARS-CoV-2 envelope gene. Based on the premise that the negative-sense replication intermediary is only present with active replication and rapidly degraded otherwise, the detection of negative-sense RNA was assessed for samples with a variety of standard RT-PCR Ct values. Detection of minus-strand RNA was associated with lower Ct value from the standard RT-PCR and was not detected in samples with high Ct values (>33). In a small fraction of samples, negative-sense RNA was detected in specimens from patients beyond the recommended time-based clearance window, suggesting that some patients may harbor actively replicating and potentially infectious virus for an extended period. This finding was corroborated in a small case series, whereby 2 patients remained SARS-CoV-2-positive for an extended period as measured by several testing modalities, including negative-sense RNA RT-PCR, sgRNA RT-PCR, and viral culture.[18] Although the presence of sgRNA or negative-sense RNA may provide an additional data point in a comprehensive risk assessment of transmission, further studies are needed to evaluate how the results, both positive and negative, from sgRNA and negative-sense RNA assays, correlate with and predict for the infectious potential of patients with SARS-CoV-2.

NEXT-GENERATION SEQUENCING

Although NGS as a technology was not new to the clinical laboratory during the COVID-19 pandemic, the diverse applications and impact deserve mention. NGS contributed to the identification and public sharing of the first SARS-CoV-2 genome, providing the global audience with the genetic sequence needed to develop targeted assays to detect the virus.[22] Since then, generation and sharing of SARS-CoV-2 genomes have occurred at an unprecedented scale, with nearly 7 million submissions to GISAID at the end of 2021. These data have allowed exceptional insight into the shifting genomic characteristics of the virus around the globe. Benefits to robust, publicly accessible sequence data include quality assurance assessment of how emerging mutations impact primer/probe binding sites by clinical laboratories,[23–25] assay manufacturers, and Food and Drug Administration (https://www.fda.gov/medical-devices/coronavirus-covid-19-and-medical-devices/sars-cov-2-viral-mutations-impact-covid-19-tests, accessed 22 September 2021). Although mutations altering test performance have been infrequent, continued vigilance is warranted and made possible through broad genomic surveillance. NGS has also allowed outbreak and epidemiologic investigations. Examples include analysis of clustered infections to highlight superspreader events,[26] evaluation of SARS-CoV-2 reinfections,[27,28] genomic data to shed light on mutations that may impact vaccine efficacy,[29] and studies showing how persistent infection can lead to variant emergence.[30] As mentioned previously, NGS has allowed the recognition of emerging variants with significant public health implications, classification as variants of interest or variants or concern (https://www.cdc.gov/coronavirus/2019-ncov/variants/variant-info.html, https://www.who.int/en/activities/tracking-SARS-CoV-2-variants/, accessed 22 September 2021), and the ability to track variant emergence and spread throughout the world using sites such as Covariants.org and Outbreak.info. The emergence of Omicron again put variant recognition and tracking on the world stage. Following initial detection, public reporting of the new variant allowed rapid assessment around the globe, tracking spread in near real time.[31] Within days, multiple countries reported cases and in the coming weeks were able to illustrate Omicron's full displacement of Delta. With potential impact to public health, laboratory diagnostics, mitigation strategies, and clinical therapeutics, continued SARS-CoV-2 genomic surveillance remains a necessity. Although high-throughput, nonclinical whole-genome sequencing has not previously been a priority for clinical laboratories, clinical laboratory leaders should lend their expertise to sequencing cores or academic laboratories capable of sustaining SARS-CoV-2 genomic sequencing efforts.[32] Beyond the genomic sequence applications, several NGS-based assays have received emergency use authorization approval as targeted diagnostics. A variety of workflows have been described using Illumina and Oxford Nanopore Technologies sequencing platforms.

CLUSTERED REGULARLY INTERSPACED SHORT PALINDROMIC REPEATS-ASSOCIATED–BASED DIAGNOSTIC TESTING FOR SEVERE ACUTE RESPIRATORY SYNDROME CORONAVIRUS 2

CRISPR (clustered regularly interspaced short palindromic repeats) RNAs (crRNAs) and Cas (CRISPR associated) nucleases function in bacteria as a form of adaptive immunity (crRNA sequences are adaptable to new threats) wherein crRNAs from the bacterial host bind target nucleic acid sequences from foreign sources and initiate Cas-mediated hydrolysis of the nucleic acids, and for some Cas nucleases, once activated, promiscuous cleavage of adjacent nucleic acids nonspecifically. CRISPR-Cas systems have been become powerful tools used to manipulate genetic material[33] and have recently been applied to diagnostic testing, taking advantage of their sequence-specific activation to provide a detection signal for microorganism nucleic acid,[34] typically following amplification by previously established methods, such as loop mediated amplification (LAMP), recombinase polymerase amplification (RPA), or PCR. Different Cas proteins operate on different nucleic acid complexes, for example, Cas 12a hydrolyzes double-stranded DNA and thus requires a reverse transcription phase for SARS-CoV-2,[35] whereas Cas 13a targets ssRNA and can be used in a direct detection application for SARS-CoV-2.[36]

Diagnostic assays using LAMP, RPA, and various flavors of PCR have existed for some time and constitute core technologies used in both commercially available and laboratory-developed tests for infectious diseases, using signal detection methods other than CRISPR-Cas systems. Although CRISPR-Cas systems do not amplify the target nucleic acid, a potential advantage of CRISPR-Cas in the detection phase is that some Cas nucleases produce signal amplification in that they can produce multiple signal molecule events per sequence-specific binding event. When coupled with a priming amplification phase, it may be possible to modestly improve on the limit of detection relative to standard molecular assays for SARS-CoV-2,[35,37] but in existing studies, the limit of detection is still similar to PCR and thus not likely to offer a meaningful difference in clinical sensitivity. Most studies evaluating CRISPR-Cas diagnostic applications use a paired amplification assay as described above, but to move CRISPR-Cas assays to the point of care and potentially reduce assay expense, it is possible to develop assays that use CRISPR-Cas detection directly on specimens with no nucleic acid extraction, and no preamplification.[36] Although there is some signal amplification, the lack of nucleic acid amplification does leave this approach with considerably higher limits of detection ($>100\times$) relative to RT-PCR, which could considerably impact the clinical sensitivity of SARS-CoV-2 assays depending somewhat on the population tested and application.[38] Like some other molecular methodologies, CRISPR-Cas assays are amenable to scale up for high-throughput application and may perform well for SARS-CoV-2 without nucleic acid extraction procedures.[39] Although CRISPR-Cas technology offers the potential for signal boosting to modestly improve the limit of detection for compatible SARS-CoV-2 testing methodologies, and is also amenable to use for direct detection when sufficient target sequence is expected in specimens, it does not appear at this time that these types of applications will lead to significant improvement in test performance characteristics relative to RT-PCR and other established methods.

MICROFLUIDIC ASSAYS FOR SEVERE ACUTE RESPIRATORY SYNDROME CORONAVIRUS 2

Microfluidic devices essentially take advantage of the physical properties of fluids to direct or even manipulate the movement of fluid specimens through engineered microchannels or material substrates. These processes may naturally separate or concentrate an analyte of interest or may be made to do so by applying an electrical charge. Lateral flow assays are a very simplistic variety of microfluidic device, and commonly used and familiar to clinical microbiologists, but there are far more sophisticated device designs as well, and different microfluidic device designs have been evaluated for developing inexpensive diagnostic tests that require no, or less, equipment than standard types of diagnostic assays.[40,41] The authors limit further discussion here to microfluidic devices evaluated with molecular SARS-CoV-2 diagnostic assays.

Isotachophoresis (ITP), a method using electrophoresis to separate and concentrate charged analytes, was used in early 2020 to develop a novel microfluidic SARS-CoV-2 detection assay.[42] ITP helped perform nucleic acid extraction and concentration with limited reagent requirements, followed by off-chip LAMP and returning to the microfluidic device for small-volume (0.2 μL) CRISPR-based detection phase in less than 30 minutes from start to finish. In a limited sample set, this test had relatively good positive percent agreement (94%) compared with a standard RT-PCR assay. Although the transition on and off chip for different phases does not result in an assay that would be appealing in its current form, this study was a technical achievement and demonstrates the potential to use ITP in a microfluidic device to reduce sample handling and dramatically reduce reagent requirements.

DISCLOSURE

The authors have nothing to disclose.

REFERENCES

1. Griesemer SB, Van Slyke G, St George K. Assessment of sample pooling for clinical SARS-CoV-2 testing. J Clin Microbiol 2021;59(4). https://doi.org/10.1128/JCM.01261-20.
2. Abdalhamid B, Bilder CR, McCutchen EL, et al. Assessment of specimen pooling to conserve SARS CoV-2 testing resources. Am J Clin Pathol 2020;153(6):715–8.
3. Smyrlaki I, Ekman M, Lentini A, et al. Massive and rapid COVID-19 testing is feasible by extraction-free SARS-CoV-2 RT-PCR. Nat Commun 2020;11(1):4812.
4. Dumm RE, Elkan M, Fink J, et al. Implementation of an extraction-free COVID RT-PCR workflow in a pediatric hospital setting. J Appl Lab Med 2021. https://doi.org/10.1093/jalm/jfab079.
5. Duffy S. Why are RNA virus mutation rates so damn high? Plos Biol 2018;16(8):e3000003. https://doi.org/10.1371/journal.pbio.3000003.
6. Ziegler K, Steininger P, Ziegler R, et al. SARS-CoV-2 samples may escape detection because of a single point mutation in the N gene. Euro Surveill 2020;25(39). https://doi.org/10.2807/1560-7917.ES.2020.25.39.2001650.
7. Wollschlager P, Todt D, Gerlitz N, et al. SARS-CoV-2 N gene dropout and N gene Ct value shift as indicator for the presence of B.1.1.7 lineage in a commercial multiplex PCR assay. Clin Microbiol Infect 2021. https://doi.org/10.1016/j.cmi.2021.05.025.
8. Enhancing readiness for Omicron (B.1.1.529): technical brief and priority actions for member states. World Health Organization. 2021. Available at: https://www.who.int/publications/m/item/enhancing-readiness-for-omicron-(b.1.1.529)-technical-brief-and-priority-actions-for-member-states.
9. Implications of the emergence and spread of the SARS-CoV-2 B.1.1. 529 variant of concern (Omicron) for the EU/EEA. European Center for Disease Prevention and Control. 2021. Available at: https://www.ecdc.europa.eu/sites/default/files/documents/Implications-emergence-spread-SARS-CoV-2%20B.1.1.529-variant-concern-Omicron-for-the-EU-EEA-Nov2021.pdf.
10. Vogels CBF, Breban MI, Ott IM, et al. Multiplex qPCR discriminates variants of concern to enhance global surveillance of SARS-CoV-2. Plos Biol 2021;19(5):e3001236.
11. Aydillo T, Gonzalez-Reiche AS, Aslam S, et al. Shedding of viable SARS-CoV-2 after immunosuppressive therapy for cancer. N Engl J Med 2020;383(26):2586–8.
12. Binnicker MJ. Can testing predict SARS-CoV-2 infectivity? The potential for certain methods to be a surrogate for replication-competent virus. J Clin Microbiol 2021;4:JCM0046921. https://doi.org/10.1128/JCM.00469-21.
13. Wolfel R, Corman VM, Guggemos W, et al. Virological assessment of hospitalized patients with COVID-2019. Nature 2020;581(7809):465–9.

14. Corbett KS, Flynn B, Foulds KE, et al. Evaluation of the mRNA-1273 vaccine against SARS-CoV-2 in nonhuman primates. N Engl J Med 2020;383(16): 1544–55.

15. Perera R, Tso E, Tsang OTY, et al. SARS-CoV-2 virus culture and subgenomic RNA for respiratory specimens from patients with mild coronavirus disease. Emerg Infect Dis 2020;26(11):2701–4.

16. van Doremalen N, Lambe T, Spencer A, et al. ChAdOx1 nCoV-19 vaccine prevents SARS-CoV-2 pneumonia in rhesus macaques. Nature 2020;586(7830): 578–82.

17. Yu J, Tostanoski LH, Peter L, et al. DNA vaccine protection against SARS-CoV-2 in rhesus macaques. Science 2020;369(6505):806–11.

18. Truong TT, Ryutov A, Pandey U, et al. Increased viral variants in children and young adults with impaired humoral immunity and persistent SARS-CoV-2 infection: a consecutive case series. EBioMedicine 2021;67:103355. https://doi.org/10.1016/j.ebiom.2021.103355.

19. van Kampen JJA, van de Vijver D, Fraaij PLA, et al. Duration and key determinants of infectious virus shedding in hospitalized patients with coronavirus disease-2019 (COVID-19). Nat Commun 2021;12(1):267.

20. Alexandersen S, Chamings A, Bhatta TR. SARS-CoV-2 genomic and subgenomic RNAs in diagnostic samples are not an indicator of active replication. Nat Commun 2020;11(1):6059.

21. Hogan CA, Huang C, Sahoo MK, et al. Strand-specific reverse transcription PCR for detection of replicating SARS-CoV-2. Emerg Infect Dis 2021;27(2):632–5.

22. Zhu N, Zhang D, Wang W, et al. A novel coronavirus from patients with pneumonia in China, 2019. N Engl J Med 2020;382(8):727–33.

23. Vanaerschot M, Mann SA, Webber JT, et al. Identification of a polymorphism in the N gene of SARS-CoV-2 that adversely impacts detection by reverse transcription-PCR. J Clin Microbiol 2020;59(1). https://doi.org/10.1128/JCM.02369-20.

24. Leelawong M, Mitchell SL, Fowler RC, et al. SARS-CoV-2 N gene mutations impact detection by clinical molecular diagnostics: reports in two cities in the United States. Diagn Microbiol Infect Dis 2021;101(3):115468.

25. Tahan S, Parikh BA, Droit L, et al. SARS-CoV-2 E gene variant alters analytical sensitivity characteristics of viral detection using a commercial reverse transcription-PCR assay. J Clin Microbiol 2021;59(7):e0007521. https://doi.org/10.1128/JCM.00075-21.

26. Lemieux JE, Siddle KJ, Shaw BM, et al. Phylogenetic analysis of SARS-CoV-2 in Boston highlights the impact of superspreading events. Sci 2021;371(6529).

27. Harrington D, Kele B, Pereira S, et al. Confirmed reinfection with SARS-CoV-2 variant VOC-202012/01. Clin Infect Dis 2021. https://doi.org/10.1093/cid/ciab014.

28. Lee JS, Kim SY, Kim TS, et al. Evidence of severe acute respiratory syndrome coronavirus 2 reinfection after recovery from mild coronavirus disease 2019. Clin Infect Dis 2020. https://doi.org/10.1093/cid/ciaa1421.

29. Hacisuleyman E, Hale C, Saito Y, et al. Vaccine breakthrough infections with SARS-CoV-2 variants. N Engl J Med 2021;384(23):2212–8.

30. Choi B, Choudhary MC, Regan J, et al. Persistence and evolution of SARS-CoV-2 in an immunocompromised host. N Engl J Med 2020;383(23):2291–3.

31. New COVID-19 variant detected in South Africa. National Institute for Communicable Diseases (NICD). 2021. Available at: https://www.nicd.ac.za/new-covid-19-variant-detected-in-south-africa/.

32. Wang J, Hawken SE, Jones CD, et al. Collaboration between clinical and academic laboratories for sequencing SARS-CoV-2 genomes. J Clin Microbiol 2022;JCM0128821. https://doi.org/10.1128/JCM.01288-21.
33. Knott GJ, Doudna JA. CRISPR-Cas guides the future of genetic engineering. Science 2018;361(6405):866–9.
34. Gootenberg JS, Abudayyeh OO, Lee JW, et al. Nucleic acid detection with CRISPR-Cas13a/C2c2. Science 2017;356(6336):438–42.
35. Joung J, Ladha A, Saito M, et al. Detection of SARS-CoV-2 with SHERLOCK one-pot testing. N Engl J Med 2020;383(15):1492–4.
36. Fozouni P, Son S, Diaz de Leon Derby M, et al. Amplification-free detection of SARS-CoV-2 with CRISPR-Cas13a and mobile phone microscopy. Cell 2021; 184(2):323–333 e9.
37. Ning B, Yu T, Zhang S, et al. A smartphone-read ultrasensitive and quantitative saliva test for COVID-19. Sci Adv 2021;7(2). https://doi.org/10.1126/sciadv.abe3703.
38. Arnaout R, Lee RA, Lee GR, et al. The limit of detection matters: the case for benchmarking severe acute respiratory syndrome coronavirus 2 testing. Clin Infect Dis 2021. https://doi.org/10.1093/cid/ciaa1382.
39. Manning BJ, Khan WA, Pena JM, et al. High-throughput CRISPR-Cas13 SARS-CoV-2 test. Clin Chem 2021;68(1):172–80.
40. Bissonnette L, Bergeron MG. Diagnosing infections–current and anticipated technologies for point-of-care diagnostics and home-based testing. Clin Microbiol Infect 2010;16(8):1044–53.
41. Chin CD, Laksanasopin T, Cheung YK, et al. Microfluidics-based diagnostics of infectious diseases in the developing world. Nat Med 2011;17(8):1015–9.
42. Ramachandran A, Huyke DA, Sharma E, et al. Electric field-driven microfluidics for rapid CRISPR-based diagnostics and its application to detection of SARS-CoV-2. Proc Natl Acad Sci U S A 2020;117(47):29518–25.